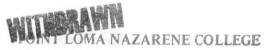

Isokinetic Exercise and Assessment

David H. Perrin, PhD, ATC
University of Virginia, Charlottesville

Human Kinetics Publishers

Library of Congress Cataloging-in-Publication Data

Perrin, David H., 1954-
    Isokinetic exercise and assessment / David H. Perrin.
      p.   cm.
    Includes index.
    ISBN 0-87322-464-7
    1. Isokinetic exercise.   I. Title.
RM727.I76P47   1993
613.7'14--dc20
                                  92-39245
                                        CIP

ISBN: 0-87322-464-7

Developmental Editor: Larret Galasyn-Wright
Managing Editor: Dawn Roselund
Assistant Editors: Valerie Hall, Julie Swadener, Moyra Knight, Laura Bofinger, and John Wentworth
Copyeditor: Chris DeVito
Proofreader: Julia Anderson
Indexer: Barbara E. Cohen
Production Director: Ernie Noa
Typesetting and Text Layout: Angela K. Snyder and Ruby Zimmerman
Text and Cover Design: Keith Blomberg
Cover Art: John W. Karapelou
Computer Graphs: Craig Ronto
Paste-Up: Tara Welsch
Printer: Versa/Dekker

Range of motion photos and overlays in Parts I and II produced by the Biomedical Communications Center of the University of Illinois at Urbana-Champaign. Other photos in Part I taken by Daniel Grogan. Isokinetic test position photos in Part II taken by Tiffany DiBlasi. Special thanks to Biodex Medical Systems, Cybex, a division of Lumex, Inc., Chattanooga Group, Inc., Loredan Biomedical Inc. and Universal Gym Equipment, Inc. for chapter 2 equipment photos.

Printed in the United States of America

10 9 8 7 6 5 4 3 2 1

Human Kinetics Publishers
Box 5076, Champaign, IL 61825-5076
1-800-747-4457

Canada:
Human Kinetics Publishers
P.O. Box 2503, Windsor, ON N8Y 4S2
1-800-465-7301 (in Canada only)

Europe:
Human Kinetics Publishers (Europe) Ltd.
P.O. Box IW14, Leeds LS16 6TR
England
0532-781708

Australia:
Human Kinetics Publishers
P.O. Box 80, Kingswood 5062
South Australia
618-374-0433

New Zealand:
Human Kinetics Publishers
P.O. Box 105-231, Auckland 1
(09) 309-2259

Betty Hale Perrin
1923–1990
From whom I learned the virtues of love,
kindness, patience, and understanding

Contents

Preface

My goal for this text is to present both the art and science of isokinetic exercise and assessment by outlining the physical, kinesiological, and physiological principles essential to understanding isokinetic theory and clinical application. With this information, clinicians and researchers can design and implement scientifically derived isokinetic test and exercise protocols.

I expect the book to be useful to practitioners, scholars, and students of rehabilitation medicine and exercise science alike. The scientific principles underlying the use of isokinetic exercise are particularly helpful to students of physical therapy, athletic training, and strength and conditioning in establishing a philosophy for clinical practice. The principles will also help physical therapists, athletic trainers, exercise physiologists, and biomechanists obtain valid and reliable quantifications of human muscle performance. The text is also a useful reference to a comprehensive list of scientifically derived normative isokinetic data in a variety of sedentary and athletic populations, both female and male and over a full range of ages.

In a brief introduction I define isokinetic resistance and compare it to isometric and isotonic modes of contraction. Part I then consists of four chapters that provide a theoretical basis for the isokinetic concept of exercise. In chapter 1 I establish appropriate terminology and describe interpretation of the normal and abnormal isokinetic torque curves. Chapter 2 surveys the isokinetic instrumentation presently available. The principles necessary for reliable assessment and for designing effective exercise programs are discussed in chapter 3. Chapter 4 addresses several areas pertinent to interpreting an isokinetic evaluation and clarifies the role of isokinetics in returning a patient to activities of daily living or athletic participation.

Part II consists of three chapters devoted to the clinical aspects of isokinetic exercise and assessment of the upper and lower extremities and of the trunk. In chapter 5 I focus on the shoulder, elbow, forearm, and wrist. The hip, knee, and ankle are addressed in chapter 6. In chapter 7 I discuss the trunk. Each chapter discusses the kinesiology of the joints, and based on these principles provides guidelines for exercise and assessment. Finally, normative data and coefficients for reliability of measurement are presented for each body region discussed; these are intended to be guidelines for female and male populations ranging from sedentary to athletic and prepubescent to adult. Only data that have undergone the scrutiny of peer review are presented.

Isokinetic exercise and assessment are not a panacea for the prevention, diagnosis, and rehabilitation of all musculoskeletal injuries. Moreover, many questions remain about both isokinetic theory and its clinical application. Where appropriate, I have identified areas in need of further scientific inquiry, in hopes that readers will be stimulated to expand our existing body of knowledge.

Acknowledgments

I owe special thanks to many people for support they gave not only during the writing of this book, but also during the first decade and a half of my career, which led to the book's conceptualization and completion.

I am indebted to James McMaster, Kenneth Metz, and Kip Smith, who gave me the opportunity to embark on a career in the exciting profession of sports medicine and athletic training at the University of Pittsburgh. Also, special thanks to Dr. Metz, who supported and orchestrated the acquisition of my first isokinetic dynamometer. I have also had the opportunity to work with outstanding professionals at two distinguished institutions—especially Richard Ray, my ultimate team physician, at the University of Pittsburgh, and my current associates at the University of Virginia, Joe Gieck, Ethan Saliba, Susan Foreman, and Frank McCue. I greatly value their collegiality, support, and friendship.

I also wish to recognize the assistance of the five major manufacturers of isokinetic dynamometry, who provided timely feedback and photographic support: in particular, Ed Dunlay, Paul Camp, and Glen Meidl of Chattanooga Group, Inc.; Peter Oppedisano, Keith McCaffrey, Joe Russo, and Mary DeGraaf of Cybex, a Division of Lumex, Inc.; Steven Westing and Janice Capobianco of Loredan Biomedical Inc.; Ed Behan and Donna Erber of Biodex Medical Systems; and Maureen Szlemp of Universal Gym Equipment, Inc.

No scholar survives without the stimulation and support provided by students. I am particularly indebted to my former undergraduate students at the University of Pittsburgh and to my past and present graduate students at the University of Virginia. Particularly noteworthy with respect to the science behind this text are my former doctoral students in sports medicine at UVa—Scott Lephart, William Quillen, Craig Denegar, Byron Shenk, Barton Buxton, Ted Worrell, Laurie Tis, and Evan Hellwig.

Three individuals deserve recognition and thanks for their important role in the development and completion of this book. Rod Harter and Tina Bonci provided critical and constructive reviews that improved the scholarly nature and clinical relevance of the work. Larret Galasyn-Wright was my developmental editor at Human Kinetics Publishers; his thoughtful perspective, timely suggestions, and editorial contributions significantly improved the final product.

Finally, I wish to express my love and thanks to Dad, Ron and Sandra, Dick, and Nancy. Only through their support did I withstand the summer of '90 and thus the realization of this goal.

A Brief Introduction to Isokinetics

The accurate assessment of human muscle performance has been the objective of exercise scientists and rehabilitation therapists for many decades. Exercise scientists interested in comparing the effects of various strength and conditioning programs seek to accurately measure muscle force. Practitioners of rehabilitation medicine want to document the efficacy of therapeutic exercise in helping patients recovering from injury to the musculoskeletal system regain their strength. Athletic trainers and sport physical therapists emphasize injury prevention by identifying underlying deficits in strength and in bilateral and reciprocal muscle group strength relationships. Underscoring all these objectives is the valid and reliable quantification of the human muscle's capacity to produce force.

ASSESSMENT OF HUMAN MUSCLE PERFORMANCE

The capacity of muscle to produce force can be assessed through either a static or dynamic contraction. Isometric (static) assessment reveals the amount of tension a muscle can generate against a resistance permitting no observable joint movement. Isotonic (dynamic) strength, the application of force through all or part of a joint's range of motion, can be assessed via a concentric (shortening) or eccentric (lengthening) mode of contraction.

Isometric Assessment

Isometric strength assessment measures a muscle's maximum potential to produce static force. Early objective testing of isometric strength was

1

performed with cable tensiometry and hand grip and back lift dynamometry. The cable tensiometer, originally designed to measure the tension of aircraft control cables, was proposed and refined as a tool for measuring the strength of human muscle groups by Clarke (1948). Accurate measurement by this method depends on a number of factors, including body position, correct joint angle (that capable of generating the greatest force), and correct location of the pulling strap on the body part serving as the fulcrum. Cable tensiometry is relatively inexpensive and capable of assessing most major muscle groups.

The primary advantage of isometric resistance is that it can be used to assess strength in or to exercise a muscle group around a joint limited in motion by either pathology or bracing. Figures 1 and 2 illustrate techniques of isometric exercise for immobilized knee and shoulder joints. Isometric strength assessment and exercise are somewhat limited because they are isolated to the specific point of application within a joint's range of motion.

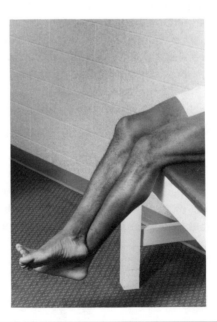

Figure 1. Use of one extremity to provide isometric resistance to the quadriceps muscles of the contralateral extremity. This resistance could be provided at different points throughout the available range of motion.

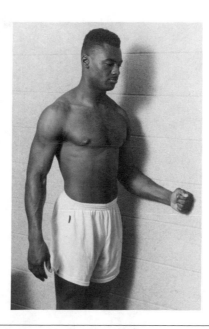

Figure 2. Use of a wall to provide isometric resistance to the shoulder external rotator muscles.

Isotonic Assessment

Isotonic strength can be measured dynamically with dumbbells, barbells, and various commercial devices. The strength of a particular muscle group is commonly determined by testing the maximum amount of weight that can be lifted through a joint's range of motion for either 1 repetition (1 RM) or 10 (10 RM). Figure 3 shows measurement of upper extremity strength using a 1-RM bench press technique with free weights. The limitations of the RM tests include the inability to control test velocity and the amount of contribution from accessory muscle groups. Moreover, isotonic resistance is limited as an exercise modality in the sense that a muscle can be overloaded only by the amount of weight that can be lifted through the weakest part of the exercised range of motion. Variable resistance equipment was designed to address this limitation; it accommodates the variations in strength by using an elliptical cam. The cam provides the least resistance where the ability to produce force is correspondingly lower (early and late in the range of motion) and the greatest resistance where the muscle is at its optimal length-tension and mechanical advantage (usually midrange).

A distinct advantage of isotonic resistance is that it permits exercise of multiple joints simultaneously. For example, the leg press (see Figure 4) exercises the quadriceps as a knee extensor and the hamstrings as a hip extensor. The resulting cocontraction may be advantageous in controlling anterior shear or displacement

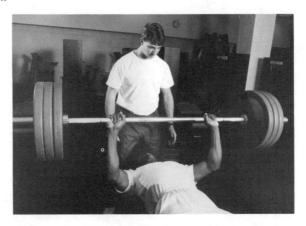

Figure 3.   Bench press to assess strength of several upper extremity muscle groups.

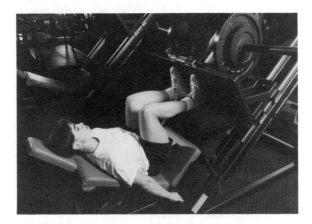

Figure 4.   Leg press to exercise several lower extremity muscle groups.

of the tibia, which would result from isolated contraction of the quadriceps muscle group. Another advantage of isotonic exercise of lower extremity muscle groups is that it may be performed in a weight-bearing or ''closed-kinetic-chain'' position. The squat exercise (see Figure 5) may be more transferable to functional weight-bearing activities of daily living and athletic participation.

Clinicians also use techniques of manual muscle testing for a gross measure of a muscle group's ability to produce force through either a static or dynamic contraction. Figures 6 and 7 illustrate manual muscle testing of upper and lower extremity muscle groups, respectively. For isometric assessment, the examiner places the joint to be tested in its midrange of motion, evenly

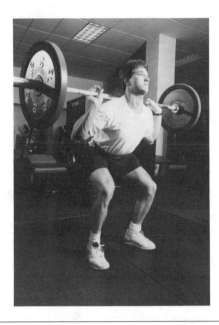

Figure 5. Squat to exercise several lower extremity muscle groups in a "closed-kinetic-chain" fashion.

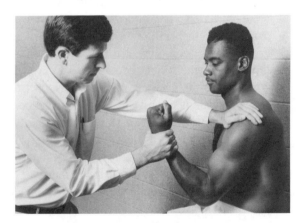

Figure 6. Manual muscle testing of the elbow flexor muscles.

matches the force produced by the patient, and subjectively grades the strength of the muscle group in question (Daniels & Worthingham, 1980; Kendall & McCreary, 1983). Isotonic assessment may be performed by noting strength as the limb moves through its available range of motion.

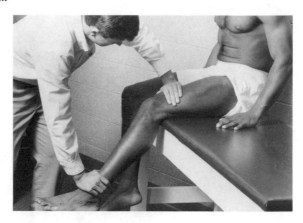

Figure 7.   Manual muscle testing of the knee extensor muscles.

Isokinetic Assessment

The concept of isokinetic exercise was developed by James Perrine and introduced in the scientific literature in 1967 by Hislop and Perrine (1967) and Thistle, Hislop, Moffroid, and Lohman (1967). Isokinetic devices allow individuals to exert as much force and angular movement as they can generate—be that large or small—up to a predetermined velocity. When a limb's angular rate of movement equals or exceeds the preset velocity limit, the dynamometer produces an equaling counterforce to ensure a constant movement rate. Note that the limb, rather than the muscle, is moving at a constant rate. Mathematical evidence has been presented that demonstrates that a constant rate of angular limb movement is not accompanied by a constant rate of muscle shortening (Hinson, Smith, & Funk, 1979). Hinson et al. (1979) succinctly stated that "the term isokinetics may be reserved to denote the type of muscular contraction which accompanies a constant angular rate of limb movement, rather than a constant linear rate of muscular shortening" (p. 34).

Isokinetic resistance has several advantages over other exercise modalities. One advantage is that a muscle group may be exercised to its maximum potential throughout a joint's entire range of motion. For example, at the midrange of joint motion (where a muscle is at its optimum length-tension relationship for the binding of actin and myosin and has its greatest mechanical advantage) the isokinetic dynamometer will maintain its preset velocity, and thus more force will be produced. Conversely, at the extremes of joint motion (where a muscle is at a physiological and mechanical disadvantage) the dynamometer will still maintain its preset velocity, but less force will be produced. Because there is no fixed resistance to move through the weakest point in a given arc of motion (as with isotonic exercise), isokinetic exercise facilitates a maximum voluntary force to be produced throughout the entire range of motion. Figure 8 illustrates the relationship between a joint's range of motion and production of isokinetic

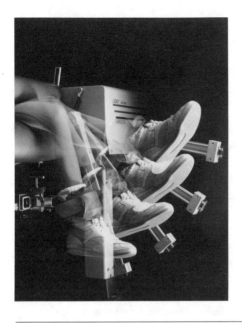
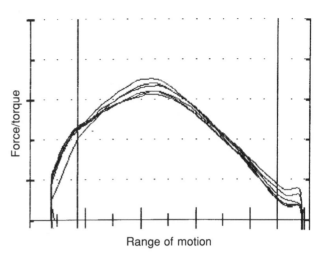

Figure 8.   Force output at the skeletal lever during isokinetic exercise. At the extremes of range the muscle has its least mechanical advantage and resistance is least. Toward midrange, where the mechanical advantage is greatest, the resistance increases proportionately.

Adapted from "The Isokinetic Concept of Exercise" by H.J. Hislop and J.J. Perrine, 1967, *Physical Therapy*, **47**, p. 116. Copyright 1967 by the American Physical Therapy Association. Adapted with the permission of the American Physical Therapy Association.

force. Figures 9 and 10 compare the force output and percentage of muscle capacity used during isotonic and isokinetic exercise, respectively.

Isokinetic resistance may also provide a safer alternative to other exercise modalities during the process of rehabilitation. Isokinetic exercise is inherently safer than isotonic because the dynamometer's resistance mechanism essentially disengages when pain or discomfort is experienced by the patient. An isokinetic apparatus may also be adapted to the particular rehabilitation challenge at hand. For example, exercise may be submaximal and easily set through pain-free ranges within the total available range of joint motion, and exercise velocities may be selected that have the least potential for joint insult.

Isokinetic exercise may be used to quantify a muscle group's ability to generate torque or force, and it is also useful as an exercise modality in the restoration of a muscle group's preinjury level of strength.

Thousands of abstracts and articles dealing with various aspects of isokinetic exercise have appeared in the scientific literature over the past 25 years. Thistle et al. (1967) were indeed prophetic when they stated, "Accommodating resistance exercise with its faculty for accommodating true muscle force capacity and permitting natural muscle torque curves, promises a new and fruitful approach to muscle exercise and analysis; and the isokinetic device offers many new and exciting applications in the study and understanding of kinesiology" (p. 282).

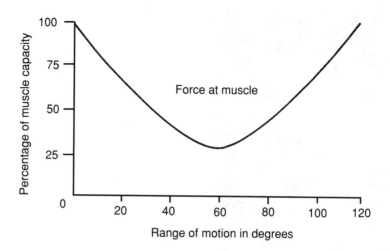

Figure 9. In isotonic exercise, resistance to the muscle varies because of the modifying effects of the lever system. Resistance has its greatest mechanical advantage on the muscle at the extremes of range and consequently the load is greatest at these points. Closer to midrange the lever is most efficient and therefore the load on the muscle is proportionately less. Demands placed on the muscle are maximum only at the extremes of the range.

From ''The Isokinetic Concept of Exercise'' by H.J. Hislop and J.J. Perrine, 1967, *Physical Therapy*, **47**, p. 115. Copyright 1967 by the American Physical Therapy Association. Adapted with the permission of the American Physical Therapy Association.

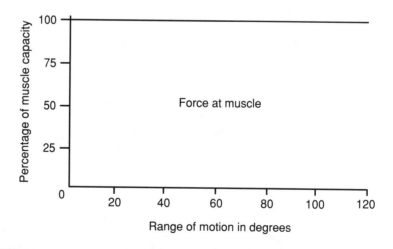

Figure 10. During isokinetic exercise the resistance accommodates the external force at the skeletal lever so that the muscle maintains maximum output throughout the full range of motion.

From ''The Isokinetic Concept of Exercise'' by H.J. Hislop and J.J. Perrine, 1967, *Physical Therapy*, **47**, p. 116. Copyright 1967 by the American Physical Therapy Association. Adapted with the permission of the American Physical Therapy Association.

Comparison of Isometric, Isotonic, and Isokinetic Exercise

Isometric

advantages
- —Useful when joint motion is contraindicated
- —Requires minimal or no equipment

disadvantages
- —Strength increases specific to exercised joint position
- —Absence of feedback from objective increases in strength

Isotonic

advantages
- —Includes a natural component of concentric and eccentric resistance
- —Positive reinforcement from progressive increases in resistance
- —Permits exercise of multiple joints simultaneously
- —Is easily performed from weight-bearing closed-kinetic-chain positions

disadvantages
- —Amount of resistance limited to weakest point in range of motion
- —Inability to quantify torque, work, and power
- —Stronger muscles may compensate for weaker muscle groups during closed-kinetic-chain exercise

Isokinetic

advantages
- —Permits isolation of weak muscle groups
- —Accommodating resistance provides maximal resistance throughout the exercised range of motion
- —Accommodating resistance provides inherent safety mechanism
- —Permits quantification of torque, work, and power

disadvantages
- —Reliable assessment is limited to isolated muscle groups through cardinal planes of motion
- —Exercise occurs primarily from non-weight-bearing open-kinetic-chain positions
- —Cost of equipment may be prohibitive for some settings

Part I

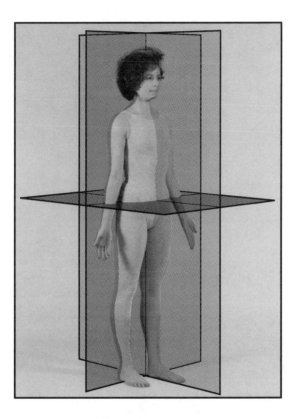

Theory of Isokinetics

Part I explains isokinetic terminology and presents an overview of each major isokinetic dynamometer currently on the market. The principles necessary for reliable assessment of human muscle performance are provided, along with the physiological rationale essential for designing an isokinetic exercise program. I also provide the key elements of a complete isokinetic assessment. You will find Part I very useful in establishing the theoretical and scientific basis necessary for the use of isokinetics in research and clinical practice.

Chapter 1

Terminology and the Isokinetic Torque Curve

A muscle can only contract or relax. When a muscle is stimulated to contract, it produces force; if this force is measured about a joint's axis of rotation, the moment of force is known as *torque*. Instruments that measure the tension produced by a muscle from the axis of rotation of a dynamometer are capable of measuring only torque. Assessment of a muscle's capacity to produce tension from the resistance pad of a dynamometer measures force, but force may be converted to torque if the distance of the resistance pad from the joint's axis of rotation is known. The SI (*Système International d'Unites*) base units or SI-derived units are the preferred method of reporting isokinetic values and are presented at the end of the chapter in Table 1.1.

AVERAGE, PEAK, AND ANGLE-SPECIFIC TORQUE

If the force or torque produced by a muscle has been assessed throughout the entire range of motion tested, the measurement may be reported as either peak or average value. The peak value would be from the point in the range of motion tested where the greatest force or torque was produced. An average value would be calculated from the tension produced by the muscle throughout the entire range of motion tested. Thus, use of average values necessitates careful standardization of the range of motion tested when making pretest, posttest, or bilateral muscle group comparisons. In contrast, peak force or torque is likely to occur within the midrange of motion assessed. As such, standardization of the range of motion tested for measurement of peak values may not be as essential as when average values are of interest. The relationship among peak and average torque and force for a given muscle contraction is quite high (see Table 1.2), suggesting that any of these values provides valid assessment of a muscle's ability to generate tension (Perrin, Tis, Hellwig, & Shenk, in press).

Peak or average torque values are the isokinetic parameters most frequently used to assess human muscle performance. However, the interfacing of microprocessors with isokinetic dynamometers enables determination of torque at any point throughout the range of motion; this is called *angle-specific torque* (AST). Although the reliability of this practice has been questioned (Kannus & Yasuda, 1992), it theoretically enables identification of torque at a predetermined point in the range of motion or a certain muscle group's contribution to the torque production.

WORK AND POWER

Isokinetic dynamometry enables the rapid and reliable quantification of force or torque. If the force and distance of a given muscle contraction are known, the amount of tension produced by the muscle may be expressed as work. If the quantity of time required to produce work is known, the ability of the muscle to generate power may be determined. Figure 1.1 illustrates peak torque, work, and power as indicated by normal isokinetic torque curves. Research has shown that the predictability of work and power from peak torque is good in both healthy and pathological knees (Kannus, 1988a, 1988b, 1988d; Kannus & Jarvinen, 1989; Morrissey, 1987). However, neuromuscular demands on upper extremity torque, work, and power within a single muscle group have not been adequately examined in the scientific literature.

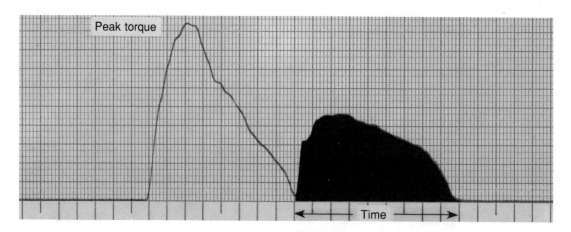

Figure 1.1 Normal isokinetic torque curves representing peak torque, work, and power. Peak torque is the single highest point of the torque curve, work is the total area under the torque curve, and power is the time required to perform work.

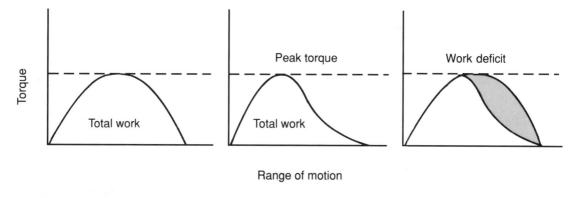

Figure 1.2 Two curves having equal values of peak torque, but an inability to produce a maximal amount of force throughout the full range of motion results in a deficit in total work in the second curve.

Moreover, the return of peak torque in a rehabilitating muscle may not be closely related to that muscle's work and power capabilities. As such, the ability to quantify torque, work, and power may be useful in both the laboratory and clinical settings. Figure 1.2 is a comparison of two torque curves having equal peak torque values, but with one producing less work than the other.

CONCENTRIC AND ECCENTRIC CONTRACTION

A muscle's ability to produce tension throughout all or part of a joint's range of motion is known as a dynamic contraction. A muscle can produce dynamic tension by either shortening or lengthening. If the joint motion is in a direction opposite the normal (gravitational) force and the tension produced by the muscle exceeds the external resistance encountered, the contraction is shortening (or concentric) in nature (Figure 1.3, a and b). If the joint motion is in the direction of the normal force and the external resistance encountered exceeds the muscle's ability to generate tension, the contraction is lengthening (or eccentric) in nature (Figure 1.4, a and b). Concentric and eccentric contractions have long been employed during isotonic exercise. More recently, the development of active dynamometry has enabled the isokinetic quantification of a muscle's ability to produce eccentric tension.

NORMAL AND ABNORMAL TORQUE CURVES

Isokinetic instruments can express muscle effort produced by a specific exercise repetition as a curve or tracing via an analog signal sent from the dynamometer. The normal concentric isokinetic torque curve is illustrated in Figure 1.5. Isokinetic resistance adjusts to the amount of force generated by a given muscle group. The combined length-tension relationship and overall effectiveness of a muscle contraction are greatest through the midrange of a joint's available range of motion and are less near the beginning and end of

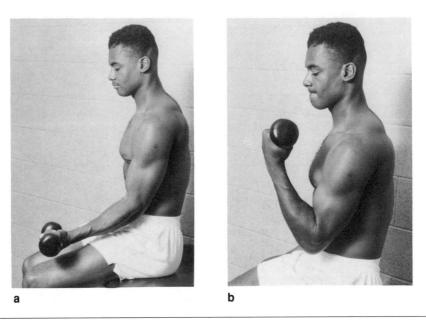

Figure 1.3 The biceps brachii and brachialis muscles before (a) and after (b) concentric (shortening) contraction.

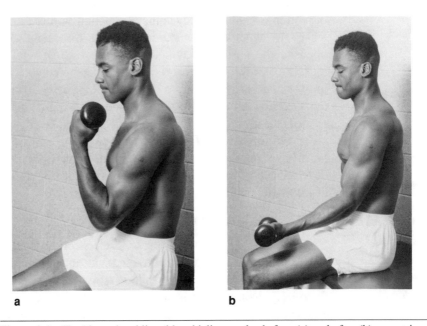

Figure 1.4 The biceps brachii and brachialis muscles before (a) and after (b) eccentric (lengthening) contraction.

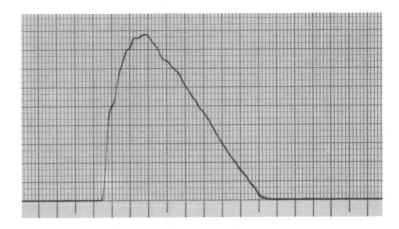

Figure 1.5   Normal concentric isokinetic torque curve. The vertical axis reflects the amount of force produced by the muscle; the horizontal axis is the range of motion through which the joint is tested.

that motion. The isokinetic torque curve reflects these variations in capacity to generate force as a muscle contracts throughout a joint's range of motion.

The torque curve illustrated in Figure 1.5 is a result of an isokinetic contraction beginning from zero velocity. To avoid impulse loading and to minimize the impact of acceleration in isokinetic testing, some instrumentation employs the use of a preload force (Jensen, Warren, Laursen, & Morrissey, 1991; Stauber, 1989b; Tis, Perrin, Weltman, Ball, & Gieck, under review). The concept of preload necessitates production of a predetermined amount of force before an isokinetic contraction can be initiated. The torque curve resulting from an isokinetic contraction with a preload force is somewhat different and is illustrated in Figure 1.6, a and b.

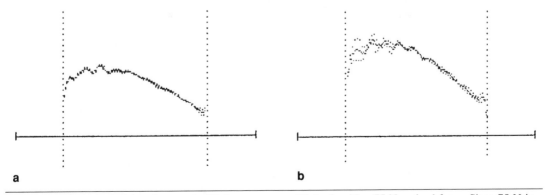

a   b

Figure 1.6   Concentric (a) and eccentric (b) force curves at 90 deg/s with a 75 N preload force. Since 75 N is required to initiate movement, the curves do not begin from the baseline.

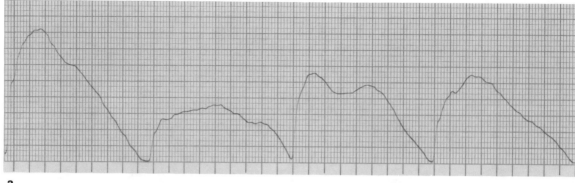

a

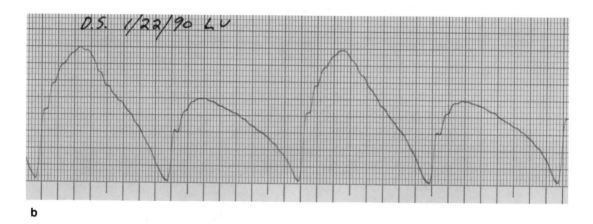

b

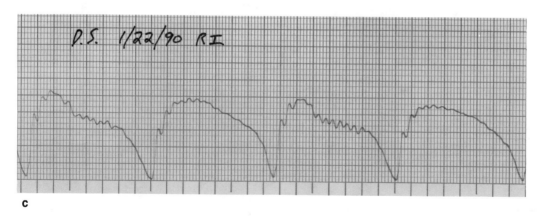

c

Figure 1.7 Torque curves resulting from a subject's attempt to feign pain during assessment of the knee extensor and flexor muscles (a). Note the inconsistent irregularities among quadriceps (1st, 3rd) and hamstring (2nd, 4th) curves. Figure 1.7b illustrates the left uninjured (LU) and (c) right injured (RI) torque curves resulting from a subject experiencing knee joint pain during isokinetic assessment. Note the consistent artifacts in the right injured (RI) torque curves for the quadriceps (1st & 3rd) contractions.

18

Several factors contribute to production of a normal, smooth, and coordinated isokinetic torque curve. The muscle group and joint being tested must be free from pain or injury. An isokinetic dynamometer accommodates pain by essentially disengaging when the patient produces less force. Pain originating from a muscle-tendon unit or from sources within an articulation crossed by a muscle group will frequently result in artifacts within the torque curve. Of special interest to a variety of clinicians has been the difficulty in replicating these artifacts from one curve to another when the muscle group or joint in question is free from pain. Figure 1.7a is an example of a subject's conscious effort to feign pain over several isokinetic contractions. The implication of this clinical observation is that an inconsistent torque curve may be useful in identifying a malingering subject. However, because this

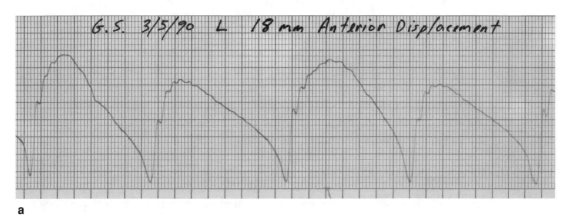

a

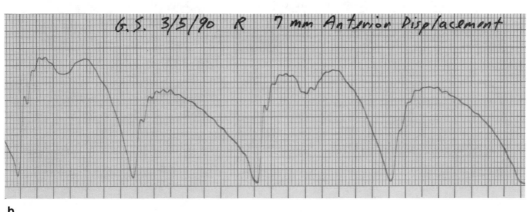

b

Figure 1.8   Torque curves produced during extension and flexion at 60 deg/s in the anterior cruciate ligament–deficient left knee (a) and uninjured right knee (b) of an intercollegiate lacrosse player. Evaluation with a KT 1000 knee arthrometer revealed 18 mm of anterior displacement in the injured left side (a) and only 7 mm of displacement in the uninjured right side (b). The injured side produced a normal torque curve while the uninjured side produced a bimodal torque curve in the absence of any appreciable amount of anterior laxity or joint pathology.

phenomenon has not been experimentally documented, conclusions about feigning based on an isokinetic torque curve should be drawn cautiously.

It has also been suggested that pathology in muscle-tendon units and bony articulations frequently shows characteristic artifacts in an isokinetic torque curve. For example, isokinetic testing of an anterior cruciate ligament–deficient knee with a distally positioned resistance pad is thought to result in a bimodal (two-peak) torque curve. The mechanism for this characteristic curve is purportedly related to the anterior translation that occurs at the proximal tibia as the quadriceps muscle group begins to contract (first peak). In the absence of an intact anterior cruciate ligament, other soft tissue structures about the knee subsequently "catch" the anterior translation of the tibia (second peak). Figure 1.8, a and b provides an example of the torque curves from an anterior cruciate ligament–deficient and normal knee of a patient in which prediction of joint pathology would obviously be questionable.

Some clinicians also claim the ability to predict a variety of other joint or muscle maladies from torque curves, including chondromalacia patella, a subluxing patella, and even a knee plica syndrome. Little or no scientific evidence exists to validate this practice. I advise clinicians to confine their interpretation of the isokinetic torque curve to a muscle's capacity to produce torque, work, and power.

INTERPRETATION OF THE TORQUE CURVE

Early isokinetic dynamometry permitted extraction of several parameters from the isokinetic torque curve including peak torque and angle-specific torques (Figure 1.9, a and b). Computerized isokinetic dynamometers now enable quantification of several additional parameters, including peak and

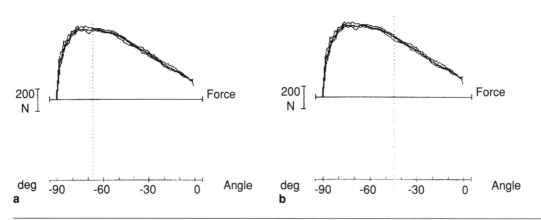

Figure 1.9 Peak torque and angle of occurrence of peak torque extrapolated from a normal curve. Angle-specific torque can be determined at any point along the curves (a and b).

average torque, peak and average force, work, and power, and extraction of several of these values from anywhere within the isokinetic torque curve. The reliability of peak torque, work, and power measures has been established for several muscle groups (Perrin, 1986). However, a large variability in the measurement of angle-specific torque has been reported (Kannus & Kaplan, 1991; Kannus & Yasuda, 1992), and the usefulness of this measure deserves further study.

One point that can be clarified at this time is the misconception that assessment of peak torque at slow isokinetic test velocities reflects strength and the torque produced at higher test velocities represents power. *Determination of torque, work, and power is independent of test velocity.*

- Torque is the force produced about a joint's axis of rotation.
- Work is the applied force times the distance of rotation.
- Power is the time required to perform work.

The capacity of a muscle to generate each of these performance parameters may be assessed at either slow, intermediate, or fast isokinetic test velocities.

Table 1.1
Systéme International d'Unites **(SI) Base Units and SI-Derived Units (With Conversion Factors)**
Pertinent to Isokinetic Assessment

	Quantity	Name of unit	Symbol
SI base units	length	meter	m
	mass	kilogram	kg
	time	second	s
SI-derived units	force	newton	N
	torque	newton meter	Nm
	work	joule	J
	power	watt	W

Conversions

Force	(lb) × 4.45 = N	(N) × .22 = (lb)
Torque	(ft-lb) × 1.36 = (Nm)	(Nm) × 0.74 = (ft-lb)
	(ft-lb) × 0.13825 = (kg-m)	(kg-m) × 7.233 = (ft-lb)
Work	(ft-lb) × .74 = (J)	(J) × 1.36 = (ft-lb)
Power	(ft-lb/s) × 1.36 = (W)	(W) × .74 = (ft-lb/s)
	(hp) × 745.7 = (W)	(W) × .0013 = (hp)
	(hp) × .17 = (kcal/s)	(kcal/s) × 5.88 = (hp)
	(ft-lb/s) × .00031 = (kcal/s)	(kcal/s) × 3234.00 = (ft-lb/s)
Angle	(deg) × .018 = (radian)	(radian) × 57.30 = (deg)
	(revolution) × 6.28 = (radian)	(radian) × .16 = (revolution)
	(deg) × .0028 = (revolution)	(revolution) × 360 = (deg)

Note. lb—pound; ft-lb—foot-pound; hp—horsepower; kcal—kilocalorie; deg—degree.

Table 1.2
Pearson Product-Moment Correlations Among Peak and Average Force and Torque of the Shoulder Internal and External Rotators

	Internal rotation average force	External rotation average force	Internal rotation peak force	External rotation peak force	Internal rotation average torque	External rotation average torque
Internal rotation peak force	.90					
External rotation peak force		.91				
Internal rotation average torque	.96		.88			
External rotation average torque		.97		.90		
Internal rotation peak torque	.86		.95		.92	
External rotation peak torque		.86		.96		.92

Note. Data from "Relationship Between Isokinetic Average Force, Peak Force, Average Torque, and Peak Torque of the Shoulder Internal and External Rotator Muscle Groups" by D.H. Perrin, L.L. Tis, E.V. Hellwig, and B.S. Shenk in press, *Isokinetics and Exercise Science.*

Chapter 2

Isokinetic Instrumentation

Not all clinical and research facilities can afford an expensive isokinetic dynamometer—I'm aware of that. But the clinician who does not have the luxury of owning a dynamometer may wish to refer a patient or athlete for isokinetic assessment to document rehabilitation progress or to obtain a preseason strength profile. Knowing the different types of dynamometers will help clinicians "shop" for a facility that can provide an isokinetic evaluation consistent with the needs of the patient or athlete in question. Figures 2.1 through 2.6 illustrate each major isokinetic dynamometer currently on the market. For those who are considering buying a dynamometer, this chapter should offer valuable education.

PASSIVE AND ACTIVE DYNAMOMETRY

Isokinetic dynamometers measure either force or torque, angular velocity, and the position of a moving body part. If a dynamometer's load cell (force- or torque-sensing apparatus) is located at the axis of rotation, the instrument measures torque. If the load cell is located distally on the resistance lever arm, the instrument measures force. In the latter case, knowing the load cell's distance from the dynamometer's axis of rotation enables the conversion of force to torque. Additionally, the software of some dynamometers calculates and reports work and power.

Dynamometers are categorized as passive or active systems (McGorry, 1989). Passive dynamometers use mechanical, magnetic, hydraulic, or electrical braking systems to dissipate force and are capable of concentric isokinetic, isotonic, or isometric modes of exercise. Active systems dissipate the force produced by a person or produce force to do work on the person. In addition to

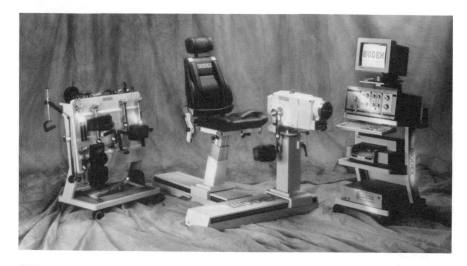

Figure 2.1   Biodex, Biodex Medical Systems, Shirley, New York.

having the capabilities of a passive system, active systems perform eccentric isokinetic and passive modes of exercise. Active systems use either an electromechanical servomotor or a hydraulic actuator as a source to perform positive work.

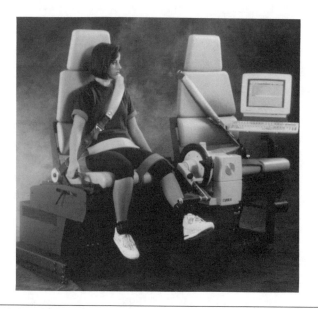

Figure 2.2   Cybex 6000, A Division of Lumex, Inc., Ronkonkoma, New York.

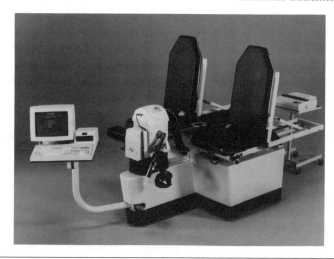

Figure 2.3   Kin-Com 500H, Chattanooga Group, Inc., Hixson, Tennessee.

Eccentric contraction has long been employed in rehabilitation and strength training via the isotonic mode of exercise. However, the ability to quantify eccentric torque, work, and power has existed only since the advent of active dynamometry in the mid-1980s. Eccentric contraction is necessary for activities of daily living and most athletic endeavors. As such, the value of assessment and exercise through both concentric and eccentric modes of contraction seems apparent (Bennett & Stauber, 1986).

Because active dynamometry produces force, it can also function as a continuous passive motion (CPM) device. CPM provides a means of imparting motion to a joint without the concomitant joint forces that occur with muscle contraction. This phenomenon may be advantageous in treating acute injuries or during postoperative rehabilitation when early motion is indicated. Research is needed to determine the usefulness of passive motion in the treatment and rehabilitation of orthopedic injuries.

COMPARISON OF ISOKINETIC EQUIPMENT

As I've explained, isokinetic dynamometers are designed as either passive or active devices. Some instruments have been of the active variety since their inception, whereas others were initially passive models and subsequently have been redesigned as active models. If assessment of both concentric and eccentric contractions is of interest, then the instrument of choice will necessarily be an active dynamometer. Other factors (in addition to cost) include range of test velocity, minimum and maximum force or torque limits, and the software's test protocol and data management capabilities.

Test Velocity

Virtually all isokinetic dynamometers can assess isometric strength, but they vary with respect to their spectrum of available test velocities beyond 0 deg/s. Some clinicians feel the capability to test through a wide spectrum of velocities is essential during both assessment and exercise. Others feel that because isokinetic exercise is a maximal form of resistance, recruitment of both slow- and fast-twitch muscle fibers may be accomplished exclusively at slower velocities. Moreover, even the fastest isokinetic velocities don't approach the angular joint velocities of many athletic activities. For example, angular velocity of the knee joint during walking and running ranges from 300 to 700 deg/s, and angular velocity of the glenohumeral joint can exceed 5,000 deg/s during baseball pitching. With respect to eccentric contraction, it should be noted that both healthy and rehabilitating individuals tend to have motor control difficulty with this form of exercise (Stauber, 1989a), particularly as test velocity increases. Anecdotal reports also exist of patients sustaining injury during high speed eccentric contractions. Perhaps the present medicolegal climate precludes the publication of these incidents of injury. If the capability to test and exercise through a wide spectrum of velocities is indeed important, it is more appropriate during concentric than eccentric isokinetic contractions. The importance of range of velocity in selecting an isokinetic dynamometer is left to the individual.

Torque Limits

Isokinetic dynamometers also are limited in the accommodating resistance they can provide. The torque limits currently available range from 250 to 500 ft-lb. When the torque limit is exceeded, a velocity error occurs or the instrument simply

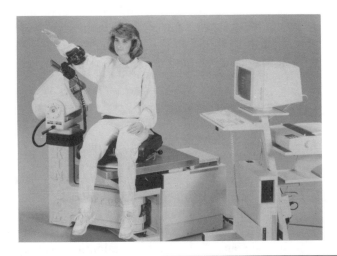

Figure 2.4   Kin-Com 125E, Chattanooga Group, Inc., Hixson, Tennessee.

shuts down. In general, lower torque limits are found in the eccentric mode of testing. These lower limits are generally adequate for testing upper extremity muscle groups, but they may not provide ample resistance when testing hip, thigh, or back musculature in healthy athletes. If your target population is primarily athletes and eccentric testing of the lower extremity is your main interest, torque limits should be carefully considered in choosing a dynamometer. But if your facility serves a wide variety of patients ranging from injured to healthy and athletic to sedentary, other features may supersede high eccentric torque limits in importance. Torque limitation is also of concern in assessment of the trunk musculature. Some isokinetic equipment includes attachments that permit exercise and assessment of trunk musculature, while other manufacturers have designed instrumentation exclusively for this purpose. Although the trunk attachments may be adequate for normal populations, the force produced by the very powerful trunk flexor and extensor muscles in some athletes may exceed the torque limits of some instruments.

Computer Software

The capabilities of a dynamometer's computer software also need your careful consideration when you compare isokinetic equipment. Some software is more conducive to collecting laboratory research data, while other software is designed primarily to meet the needs of a clinical rehabilitation facility. Software packages vary in capabilities for database management and flexibility in design of test protocols. For example, assessment of isokinetic strength of reciprocal muscle groups in a continuous concentric/concentric fashion is a desirable feature for some buyers, whereas the ability to focus on one major muscle group through concentric/eccentric modes of contraction

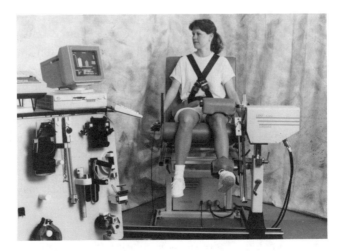

Figure 2.5   Lido, Loredan Biomedical Inc., West Sacramento, California.

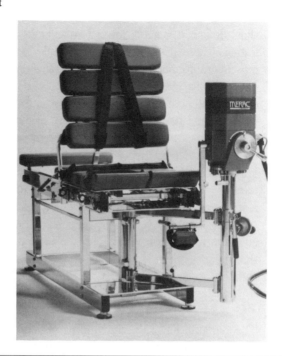

Figure 2.6   Merac, Universal Gym Equipment, Inc., Cedar Rapids, Iowa.

is important to others. The ability to quantify torque, work, and power is also important to many clinicians, and some software reports each of these isokinetic values. Other software is more versatile in extracting peak and average torque values along any or all points of each individual torque curve.

Ancillary Functions

Most instruments currently on the market fall under the category of active dynamometers, with the capacity to function in a passive mode and perhaps also isotonic and isometric modes of resistance. In theory, a dynamometer that provides continuous passive motion, isometric resistance, and isotonic and isokinetic concentric and eccentric resistance can take a patient through virtually every phase of rehabilitation. In reality, the use of a dynamometer as an exercise modality for each phase of rehabilitation is probably not cost- or time-effective in most settings. Other means exist to provide passive motion and isometric and isotonic resistance during rehabilitation. The value of an isokinetic dynamometer in performing these ancillary tasks may be overrated.

Instrument Reliability

Whatever functions you require of a dynamometer, you'll want to be assured of its reliability in measuring torque, velocity, and angular position. You can test mechanical reliability by simply hanging a known weight on the load cell of the instrument (torque) and noting the time required to move through a known distance at a specific angular velocity (velocity and angular position). Mechanical reliability has been reported in the scientific literature for several isokinetic dynamometers (Bemben, Grump, & Massey, 1988; Farrell & Richards, 1986; Patterson & Spivey, 1992; Taylor, Sanders, Howick, & Stanley, 1991).

The introduction of the human element complicates the issue of reliability for both the tester and the person being tested. You will enhance intertester and intratester reliability by adhering to established protocols, particularly with respect to patient setup and the presence or absence of verbal encouragement. Subject reliability is more complex. For example, willingness to provide maximum effort and tolerance of the discomfort of maximum muscle contraction may confound the reliability of measurement. I discuss the reliability of isokinetic dynamometry in measuring human muscle performance at the various joints in chapter 5 (upper extremity), chapter 6 (lower extremity), and chapter 7 (trunk).

Durability, warranty, and the reliability of the manufacturer's service are paramount in your choice of an isokinetic dynamometer. The warranty protection provided by each of the major manufacturers usually includes parts, labor, travel, freight, and software upgrades for 12 months. All manufacturers purport to sell and service exemplary instrumentation. Indeed, the sophistication of the dynamometers available is remarkable. But I advise you to contact several clinical and research facilities to explore the opinions of those with extensive experience with isokinetic dynamometers.

DESCRIPTION OF ISOKINETIC INSTRUMENTATION

A detailed description of each isokinetic dynamometer would make this book out of date before its first printing. Isokinetic instrumentation is undergoing continual modification and improvement, and in recent years a very competitive atmosphere has evolved among manufacturers. By providing you a summary of the major features of each dynamometer, I leave you to decide which dynamometer best meets the needs of your facility and your clientele. Table 2.1 summarizes features with respect to mode of contraction, test velocity, and torque/force limitation, and Table 2.2 gives an overview of computer specifications for each instrument.

Dynamometer	Modes	Test velocities	Torque/force limits
Biodex	Isokinetic		
	Concentric	30-450 deg/s	450 ft-lb
	Eccentric	5-150 deg/s	300 ft-lb
	Isometric	0 deg/s	450 ft-lb
	Isotonic	0-450 deg/s	300 ft-lb
	Passive	2-150 deg/s	300 ft-lb
Cybex 6000	Isokinetic		
	Powered eccentric	15-55 deg/s	250 ft-lb
		60-120 deg/s	300 ft-lb
	Powered concentric	15-300 deg/s	500 ft-lb
	Nonpowered concentric	15-500 deg/s	500 ft-lb
	CPM	60-120 deg/s	300 ft-lb
		5-55 deg/s	250 ft-lb
Kin-Com 500H	Isokinetic		
	Concentric	1-250 deg/s	455 lb
	Eccentric	1-250 deg/s	455 lb
	Isotonic		
	Concentric	1-250 deg/s	455 lb
	Eccentric	1-250 deg/s	455 lb
	Isometric	0 deg/s	455 lb
	Passive	1-250 deg/s	450 lb
Kin-Com 125E	Isokinetic		
	Concentric	1-250 deg/s	450 lb
	Eccentric	1-250 deg/s	450 lb
	Isotonic		
	Concentric	1-250 deg/s	450 lb
	Eccentric	1-250 deg/s	450 lb
	Isometric	0 deg/s	450 lb
	Passive	1-250 deg/s	22 lb
Lido	Isokinetic		
	Concentric	1-400 deg/s	400 ft-lb
	Eccentric	1-250 deg/s	250 ft-lb
	CPM	1-120 deg/s	250 ft-lb
	Isometric	0 deg/s	350 ft-lb
	Isotonic		
	Concentric	1-400 deg/s	400 ft-lb
Merac	Isokinetic		
	Concentric	15-500 deg/s	500 ft-lb
	Isotonic		
	Concentric	1-1000 deg/s	500 ft-lb
	Dynamic variable	1-1000 deg/s	500 ft-lb
	Isometric	0 deg/s	500 ft-lb

Table 2.1
Summary of Isokinetic Dynamometer Specifications

Note. CPM—continuous passive motion.

Table 2.2
Computer Specifications for the Major Isokinetic Dynamometers

Dynamometer	Computer	Hard drive	Floppy disk drive	Monitor	Printer options
Biodex	Intel 386 SX 2 Mb RAM	42 Mb	1.2 Mb 5-1/4"	VGA color	Deskjet
Cybex	Intel 386 DX 2 Mb RAM	42 Mb	1.2 Mb 5-1/4"	VGA color	Black and white or color
Kin-Com	386 SX-33 MHz 4 Mb RAM	105 Mb	40/120 Mb tape backup 3-1/2"	VGA color	Color or laserjet
Lido	Intel 386-25 MHz 2 Mb RAM	40 Mb	1.44 Mb 3-1/2"	VGA color	Black and white dot or laser
Merac	Intel 286 640 K memory	120 Mb	1.44 Mb 3-1/2"	VGA color	Dot or deskjet

Note. Mb—megabite; RAM—random access memory; MHz—megahertz; K—kilobite; VGA—Video Graphics Adaptor.

Chapter 3

Principles of Isokinetic Testing and Exercise

Factors that confound the accurate and reliable assessment of human muscle performance deserve careful attention in the development of standard test protocols. Indeed, any isokinetic evaluation should be preceded by a thorough screening of the musculoskeletal region to be tested. Patients experiencing a muscle in spasm or a joint restricted in motion by inflammation, effusion, or muscle contracture are not candidates for isokinetic assessment or exercise. Moreover, individuals at risk for cardiovascular problems (e.g., those who are obese or severely deconditioned; sedentary men over 40 years old or sedentary women over 50) should be carefully screened before undergoing evaluation involving vigorous exercise (American College of Sports Medicine, 1991). Evidence has also been presented that patients receiving anticoagulant therapy for cerebral, cardiac, or venous reasons may be at risk of hemorrhagic complications during isokinetic exercise (Richter, 1992). The following principles should be considered once the determination has been made to proceed with isokinetic assessment or exercise.

PATIENT EDUCATION, FAMILIARIZATION, AND WARM-UP

Isokinetic resistance is a novel sensation. You can attain reliable and valid assessment only with adequate patient education and familiarization with the isokinetic concept of exercise. You need to advise patients that an isokinetic dynamometer is set at a predetermined velocity and that resistance will be encountered only when the patient attempts to move the body segment at an equal or greater velocity. In short, the dynamometer's function is to dissipate energy produced by the patient. Instruct patients to "push and pull as hard and fast as you can." The advent of active isokinetic dynamometry now enables assessment and exercise through eccentric as well as concentric modes of contraction. This capability requires additional education of and familiarization by patients because dynamometers can apply force. Inform your patients that the instrument will attempt to "push or pull" their limb (eccentric contraction), and that they should resist the movement of the lever arm.

In the case of both concentric and eccentric contraction, an adequate familiarization period should be provided for each patient in the form of warm-up repetitions prior to assessment at each test velocity, and should consist of first submaximal and then maximal efforts. In general, three submaximal and three maximal repetitions are adequate to obtain reliable measurements of isokinetic peak torque, work, and power (Perrin, 1986).

BODY POSITION, STABILIZATION, AND JOINT ALIGNMENT

Position and stabilize patients on a dynamometer in a manner designed to isolate the target muscle group and to eliminate (as much as possible) contribution from accessory muscle groups. With this goal in mind, you should stabilize subjects with straps at both the waist and chest. To eliminate contribution from the upper extremities during assessment of a lower extremity muscle group, the subject's arms should be placed across the chest. Similarly, the feet should be in a non-weight-bearing position during assessment of upper extremity muscle groups. Figure 3.1 illustrates the classic seated test position for the knee and Figure 3.2 is a recommended position for assessment of shoulder rotation strength.

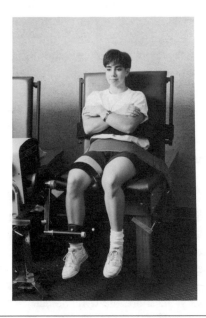

Figure 3.1   Classic seated knee test position with body stabilized by straps around thigh, waist, and chest, and with arms folded across chest.

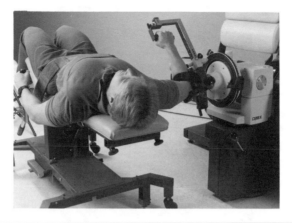

Figure 3.2   Supine test position for assessment of shoulder rotator muscles with body stabilized by straps around waist and chest.

In order to isolate the performance of single muscle groups, isokinetic testing usually occurs through the cardinal planes of the body (Figure 3.3). These movements and planes include flexion and extension through the sagittal plane, abduction and adduction through the frontal plane, and rotation through the transverse plane (Figures 3.4, a and b-3.6, a and b). To facilitate movement through these planes, the axis of rotation of the joint being assessed should be aligned as closely as possible with the axis of rotation of the test or exercise

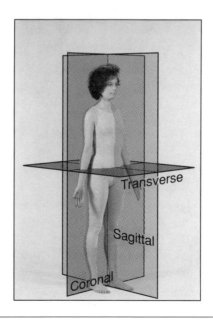

Figure 3.3   Cardinal planes of the body.

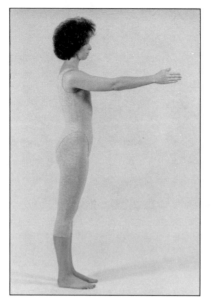
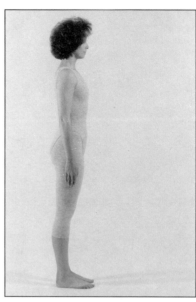

a   b

Figure 3.4 Flexion (a) and extension (b) of the glenohumeral joint through the sagittal plane.

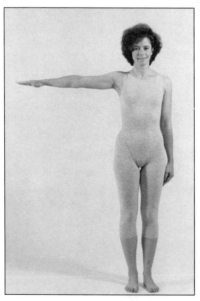
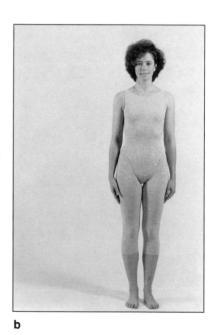

a   b

Figure 3.5 Abduction (a) and adduction (b) of the glenohumeral joint through the frontal (coronal) plane.

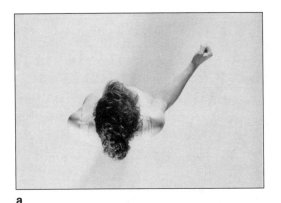   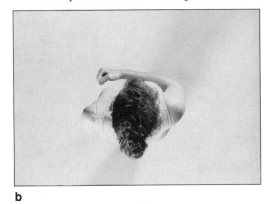

a   b

Figure 3.6   External (a) and internal (b) rotation of the glenohumeral joint through the transverse plane.

dynamometer. Although the instantaneous center of rotation of the joint constantly changes during joint motion, passive movement through the range of motion to be tested prior to actual assessment is useful in assuring proper joint and dynamometer alignment and correct lever-arm length.

GRAVITY CORRECTION

When isokinetic assessment involves movement of a limb through a gravity-dependent position, you should employ gravity correction procedures to account for the weight of the dynamometer's lever arm and the limb being tested (Figures 3.7 & 3.8). Regardless of muscle group, acceleration of the limb due to gravity erroneously adds to torque. Conversely, additional force must be exerted to accelerate the limb against gravity, and this tends to reduce the torque output recorded. The importance of gravity correction in obtaining valid strength measures, particularly of the quadriceps and hamstring muscle groups, has been established (Bohannon & Smith, 1989; Perrin, Haskvitz, & Weltman, 1991; Rothstein, Lamb, & Mayhew, 1987; Winter, Wells, & Orr, 1981). In the case of the thigh musculature, quadriceps force may be underpredicted by 4% to 43%, and hamstring force may be overpredicted by 15% to 510% (Nelson & Duncan, 1983; Winter et al., 1981). When shoulder internal and external rotation are assessed from a seated position, the internal rotators are assisted by gravity and the external rotators are opposed by gravity. Gravity correction tends to increase values obtained during shoulder external rotation and decrease values obtained during internal rotation.

Failure to correct for the effects of gravity also confounds determination of reciprocal muscle group ratios. For example, because gravity correction tends to reduce hamstring force and increase quadriceps force, determination of the hamstring/quadriceps reciprocal muscle group ratio from uncorrected values tends to inflate the ratio (Figoni, Christ, & Massey, 1988; Fillyaw, Bevins, &

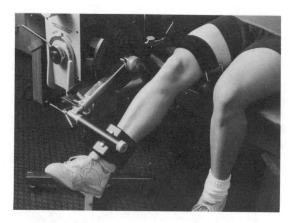

Figure 3.7   Assessment of knee extensor and flexor muscles from a gravity-dependent position. Gravity correction would add to quadriceps torque and subtract from hamstring torque.

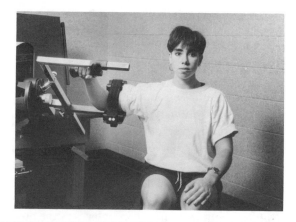

Figure 3.8   Assessment of shoulder internal and external rotator muscles from a gravity-dependent position. Gravity correction would add to external rotator torque and subtract from internal rotator torque.

Fernandez, 1986). In other words, the hamstring muscle group would appear to be stronger relative to the quadriceps muscle group than is actually the case. A similar phenomenon exists for the reciprocal muscle group ratio for the shoulder external and internal rotators. Gravity correction appropriately increases shoulder external rotation values and decreases internal rotation values, thereby increasing the external/internal rotation reciprocal muscle group ratio; in some cases to the point where the external rotators are actually stronger than the internal rotators (Perrin, Hellwig, Tis, & Shenk, 1992) (Figure 3.9).

It is clear that gravity correction influences strength and reciprocal muscle group ratios of the lower and upper extremities. I recommend gravity cor-

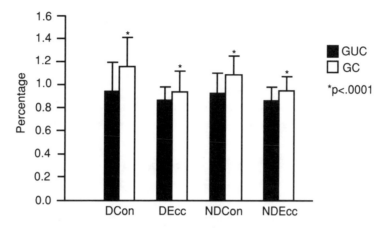

Figure 3.9   Gravity uncorrected (GUC) and gravity corrected (GC) shoulder external/internal rotation reciprocal muscle group ratios determined from dominant (D) and nondominant (ND) side concentric (Con) and eccentric (Ecc) average force values. Gravity correction added to external rotation average force and subtracted from internal rotation average force. * indicates GC values greater than GUC values.

From "Effect of Gravity Correction on Shoulder Rotation Isokinetic Average Force and Reciprocal Muscle Group Ratios" by D.H. Perrin, E.V. Hellwig, L.L. Tis, and B.S. Shenk, 1992, *Isokinetics and Exercise Science*, **2**, p. 32.

rection procedures for assessment of any muscle group where movement is aided or resisted by the effect of gravity. Appropriate reporting of isokinetic data requires explanation of test position and a description of the gravity correction procedure employed. Only in this way can you be assured of appropriate interpretation and replication of isokinetic test protocols.

Although gravity correction is important in the valid assessment of many muscle groups of the trunk and extremities, it may confound comparison of bilateral strength relationships between extremities and interpretation of any changes in strength found during subsequent evaluations. For example, if an error is made in the gravity correction procedure when testing a contralateral extremity, any differences could be related to the magnitude of the different gravity correction factor rather than to true differences between extremities. Moreover, if an independent gravity correction procedure is used in a test and retest situation, any changes in strength may be due to a training effect or to a different gravity correction factor. The reliability of the gravity correction procedure becomes essential during any retest sessions. Indeed, I recommend that you use the same gravity correction factor (via computer software or lever-arm manipulation) obtained during the initial test session during any subsequent evaluations in either clinical or laboratory settings. The exceptions to this recommendation would be if a significant amount of muscle atrophy existed in the injured extremity during the initial test session, or if substantial increases in a healthy muscle's cross-sectional area were expected to result from a training program. When making bilateral comparisons between extremities, again use an identical gravity correction factor unless one of the tested extremities has a substantial amount of muscle atrophy. Additional research is needed to determine the reliability of the gravity correction procedure on each of the existing isokinetic dynamometers and its role in test-retest strength assessment.

THE "OVERSHOOT" PHENOMENON

Engaging an isokinetic dynamometer's resistance mechanism necessitates accelerating a limb to a predetermined test velocity. Deceleration of the overspeeding limb and lever arm produces a transient peak, or spike, in the isokinetic torque curve: This is the "overshoot" phenomenon (Sapega, Nicholas, Sokolow, & Saraniti, 1982). Figure 3.10, a and b illustrates the overshoot curve that results from undamped and damped isokinetic torque tests. Determining peak values from the artificial spike may confound interpretation of a muscle's true capacity to produce maximal force. To compensate for this deceleration mechanism, various isokinetic manufacturers have incorporated a "damp," "ramp," or "preload" feature into their instrumentation. More recently, "isoacceleration" has been introduced; this preprograms the rate of acceleration and deceleration during resistive exercise (Seger, Westing, Hanson, Karson, & Ekblom, 1988; Westing, Seger, & Thorstensson, 1991).

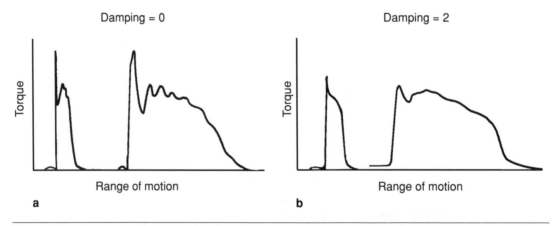

Figure 3.10   Two curves illustrating the effect of damping on torque "overshoot" (a and b). A damping of 2 reduces the amount of artifact that could incorrectly be interpreted at peak torque (b).
From "The Nature of Torque 'Overshoot' in Cybex Isokinetic Dynamometry" by A.A. Sapega, J.A. Nicholas, D. Sokolow, and A. Saraniti, 1982, *Medicine and Science in Sports and Exercise,* **14**(5), p. 368. Copyright 1982 by The American College of Sports Medicine. Reprinted by permission.

Damping is a method of reducing overshoot and is used to facilitate identification of torque that is free from artifacts and peak torque overshoot (Sinacore, Rothstein, Delitto, & Rose, 1983). In general, a larger damping setting is indicated where greater amounts of force are required to decelerate an overspeeding lever arm-limb unit. The greater the force produced at slow concentric isokinetic velocities, the greater the damping setting. Similarly, greater levels of preload force are indicated where larger and stronger muscle groups are being tested. As with gravity correction, you should report the respective damping or preload procedures employed during isokinetic testing.

It is important to recognize that damping influences the torque curve relative to the time base (Rothstein et al., 1987). In other words, damping causes a shift in the torque curve relative to range of motion. Thus, measurement of angle-specific torque is confounded by the damping setting, with the amount of inaccuracy dependent on the amount of damping. Accurate determination of angle-specific torque requires using a damping setting of zero (Sinacore et al., 1983).

In addition, although damping is intended to eliminate artifacts or peak torque overshoot, it has the potential to eliminate some aspect of the torque signal itself. Moreover, the exact changes in the analog torque curve due to damping are unknown and thus unquantifiable. More recently, some instrumentation has introduced the concept of "ramping," which is designed to control the rate of acceleration. This feature may be more desirable than damping.

Static preloading requires that a predetermined force be produced by the subject before movement is permitted by the dynamometer (Jensen et al., 1991). As with damping, use of high or low preload conditions will affect interpretation of the isokinetic torque curve. For example, use of a high preload condition requires a muscle to generate a considerable amount of tension before motion will begin, so higher levels of torque will be recorded earlier in the range of motion than under a low preload condition. The average torque produced by the muscle will thus be greater than that produced through an equal range of motion but under a lesser preload condition. Comparison of peak torque values obtained from high and low preload conditions is not affected to the same extent as measures of average torque (Jensen et al., 1991). The enhancement of torque early in the range of motion, which is associated with a higher preload force, is the probable mechanism for the greater values of average torque found with the use of a preload force (Kramer, Vaz, & Hakansson, 1991). Figures 3.11, a and b and 3.12, a and b illustrate the concentric and eccentric torque curves produced from high and low preload conditions at two test velocities.

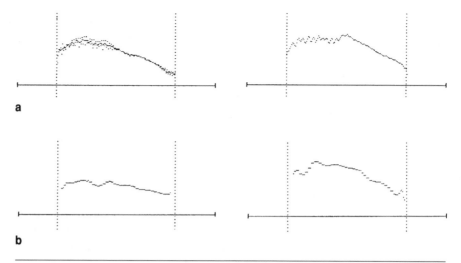

Figure 3.11 Concentric (left) and eccentric (right) force curves produced during knee extension at 30 (a) and 150 (b) deg/s with a 75 N preload.

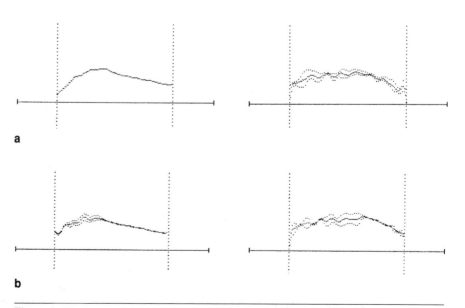

Figure 3.12 Concentric (left) and eccentric (right) force curves produced during knee extension at 90 deg/s with a 0 N (a) and 75 N (b) preload. Note that the 0 N preload curve begins closer to the baseline than the 75 N preload curve.

FACTORS CONFOUNDING ACCURATE ISOKINETIC ASSESSMENT

Determination of a muscle's maximal capacity to produce force assumes the muscle-tendon unit is intact, is receiving normal innervation from the nervous system, and is free from pain. In some cases, submaximal isokinetic exercise may be indicated to train a muscle experiencing a deficit somewhere in its neuromuscular mechanism. However, accurate identification of deficits in torque, work, or power of a single muscle group is impossible if pain is experienced by the subject during isokinetic assessment. The effect of pain on isokinetic assessment is illustrated in Figures 3.13 and 3.14, a and b. This athlete was tested to determine the status of his exercise program following several weeks of intense rehabilitation following rupture of the anterior cruciate ligament. He produced typical quadriceps and hamstring injured side isokinetic torque curves as compared to the uninjured extremity (Figure 3.13, a and b). Following 6 months of additional

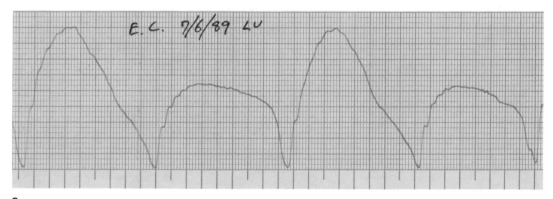

a

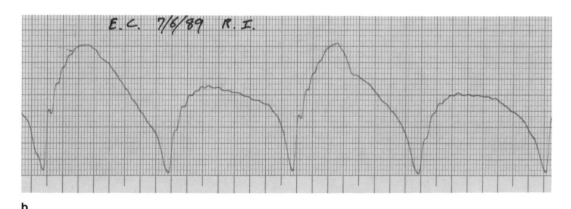

b

Figure 3.13 Left uninjured (a) and right injured (b) side torque curves of the quadriceps and hamstring muscle groups in an intercollegiate lacrosse player. Evaluation revealed only a minor deficit in injured side quadriceps peak torque. LU and RI indicate left uninjured and right injured extremities, respectively.

rehabilitation, the athlete was again assessed for isokinetic strength before being allowed to begin strenuous preseason training camp. Figure 3.14b shows an abnormal torque curve with obvious deficits in quadriceps peak torque as compared to the uninjured side (Figure 3.14a). When questioned, the athlete indicated he had just completed several days of intense exercise and had experienced pain within the knee joint during the repeat isokinetic evaluation. After several days of rest, the athlete completed an additional isokinetic evaluation that indicated normal strength in the quadriceps and hamstring muscle groups. The first repeat isokinetic assessment could have been falsely interpreted as revealing significant

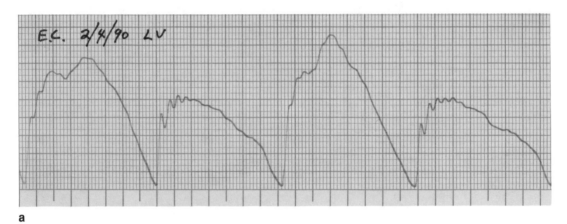

a

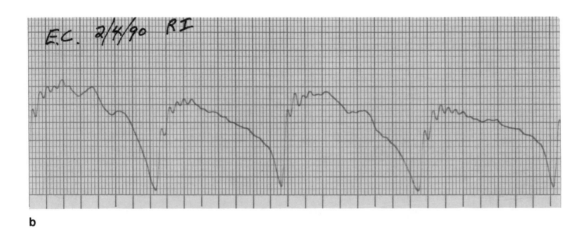

b

Figure 3.14   Follow-up evaluation of left uninjured (a) and right injured (b) side quadriceps and hamstring muscle groups of the same athlete in Figure 3.13. Evaluation revealed a significant deficit in injured side quadriceps peak torque that was a result of pain during knee extension. LU and RI indicate left uninjured and right injured extremities, respectively.

deficits in strength of the injured extremity. Regardless of the source, accurate assessment of maximal force can be accomplished only when a pain-free state exists.

Coactivation or cocontraction of an antagonist muscle group may also influence the force production of an agonist muscle group. For example, during knee extension, coactivation of the hamstring muscle group may detract from the peak torque recording of the quadriceps muscle group. Osternig, Hamill, Lander, and Robertson (1986) obtained simultaneous recordings of torque, angular displacement, and agonist/antagonist electromyographic activity of the quadriceps and hamstring muscle groups during isokinetic assessment at 100 deg/s and 400 deg/s. They reported that hamstring coactivation increased substantially during the last 25% of knee extension (Figures 3.15 and 3.16). In contrast, antagonist activity of the quadriceps muscle group remained low during knee flexion. The discrepancy between muscle groups was unclear. Further research is needed to examine the influence of coactivation of the muscle groups about a variety of joints. The influence of a test protocol that employs continuous reciprocal contractions of agonist and antagonist muscle groups and a protocol that assesses torque from repeated isolated contractions of a single muscle group also deserves further attention.

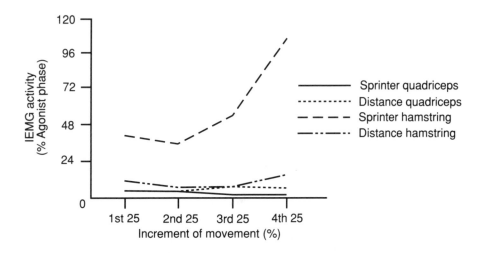

Figure 3.15   Mean IEMG (integrated electromyography) activity of antagonist quadriceps and hamstrings for first through fourth quarters of knee extension/flexion at 100 deg/s. From "Co-Activation of Sprinter and Distance Runner Muscles in Isokinetic Exercise" by L.R. Osternig, J. Hamill, J.E. Lander, and R. Robertson, 1986, *Medicine and Science in Sports and Exercise,* **18**(4), p. 434. Copyright 1986 by The American College of Sports Medicine. Reprinted by permission.

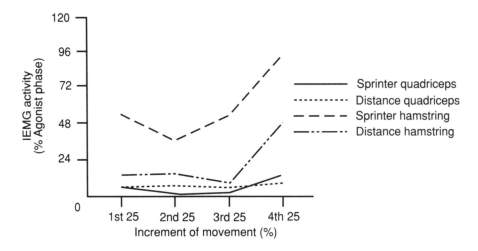

Figure 3.16   Mean IEMG (integrated electromyography) activity of antagonist quadriceps and hamstrings for first through fourth quarters of knee extension/flexion at 400 deg/s. From "Co-Activation of Sprinter and Distance Runner Muscles in Isokinetic Exercise" by L.R. Osternig, J. Hamill, J.E. Lander, and R. Robertson 1986, *Medicine and Science in Sports and Exercise,* **18**(4), p. 434. Copyright 1986 by The American College of Sports Medicine. Reprinted by permission.

TEST PROTOCOLS

A wide variety of test protocols exists for assessment of isokinetic torque, work, and power. However, several essential components should be included to obtain optimal stability and reliability of measurement.

Warm-Up

Begin each test protocol with a warm-up session that includes both submaximal and maximal repetitions. Johnson and Siegel (1978) found that three submaximal and three maximal warm-up repetitions were necessary before stability of measurement could be obtained during isokinetic assessment of knee extensor peak torque. Good reliability of measurement has also been reported using this warm-up protocol in obtaining measures of peak torque, work, and power during assessment of knee and shoulder flexion and extension and shoulder internal and external rotation (Perrin, 1986). A warm-up session should precede each isokinetic test velocity. Research has also shown that 1 or 2 days of familiarization and training before actual testing enhances reliability of isokinetic measurement (Kues, Rothstein, & Lamb, 1992).

Rest

The protocol should also provide for a consistent rest interval between each series of test repetitions and test velocities. Research has shown that an interval of rest enables production of greater amounts of isokinetic strength with higher reliability of measurement than when no rest is provided between trials (Stratford, Bruulsema, Maxwell, Black, & Harding, 1990). The amount of rest provided will depend on the nature of the test. For example, 30 seconds to 1 minute is probably sufficient for recovery after four maximal repetitions at any test velocity. However, a 25 to 30 repetition endurance test requires at least 1 minute of rest and perhaps longer, depending on the fitness level of the individual you are testing.

Test Velocity

The variations in motor unit recruitment patterns and muscle fiber composition between individuals and between muscle groups in any one individual may justify assessment and exercise through a spectrum of slow to fast isokinetic velocities. Because isokinetic resistance is a novel experience for everyone, I recommend that you test slow velocities first. This will facilitate motor learning at a slow velocity prior to testing at faster velocities (Griffin, 1987). Also, lower reliability of measurement has been reported when higher test velocities precede slower velocities in subjects that have limited experience on an isokinetic dynamometer (Wilhite, Cohen, & Wilhite, 1992).

It is a common misconception that high velocity isokinetic exercise approximates the velocity of joint movement found during many athletic activities. Peak angular velocities of shoulder internal rotation during the acceleration phase of throwing average 6,180 deg/s in professional pitchers and have been found as high as 9,198 deg/s (Pappas, Zawacki, & Sullivan, 1985). Although an extreme example, this peak angular velocity is about 18 times higher than the fastest test velocity available on a commercial isokinetic dynamometer. In reality, isokinetic exercise does not approach the functional angular velocities of joint movement found in many athletic activities.

Number of Test Repetitions

Multiple contractions are necessary to obtain a true maximal value of force or torque, regardless of test velocity. Maximum torque is typically evaluated from the first two to six contractions (Baltzopoulos & Brodie, 1989). The software of some dynamometers permits measurement of torque using a visual overlay technique. That is, each subsequent repetition is displayed as a torque curve that overlays the previous repetition. In this way, you can accept or reject each torque curve until a true maximal effort is achieved. Other software will simply record the highest value from a predetermined number of test repetitions. In either case, I recommend three to four repetitions to achieve measurement of maximum torque.

Verbal Encouragement

The presence or absence of verbal encouragement can also have a dramatic effect on ability to produce maximum effort. Encouragement is probably more likely to stimulate a maximum effort during any kind of strength assessment or performance. But because encouragement could not be consistent among testers or between test sessions, subjects should be instructed before each series of repetitions to produce a maximum effort, and the tester should remain silent during the test.

Visual Feedback

Inherent to all isokinetic dynamometry is a numerical, digital, or visual display of the patient-generated torque curve. Visual feedback, or knowledge of results during assessment, may improve a maximum voluntary contraction during an isokinetic test session. Several authors have reported greater levels of peak torque of the quadriceps and/or hamstring muscle groups when subjects were provided knowledge of results during slow speed isokinetic testing (Baltzopoulos, Williams, & Brodie, 1991; Hald & Bottjen, 1987), with increases as great as 12% at 15 deg/s (Figoni & Morris, 1984). Somewhat controversial is the impact of knowledge of results during high speed isokinetic assessment. Baltzopoulos et al. (1991) and Figoni and Morris (1984) reported no effect during assessment at 180 deg/s and 300 deg/s, respectively, while Hald and Bottjen (1987) found greater peak torque at 180 deg/s with visual feedback. The failure to see any effect during high speed testing may be due to an insufficient period of time for the central nervous system to process the visual information. Most importantly, isokinetic assessment should be consistent with respect to the presence or absence of visual feedback.

Visual feedback may also be useful to induce a greater overload during isokinetic training. Indeed, Croce (1986) found that the use of visual and auditory electromyographic (EMG) feedback during isokinetic training produced significantly greater increases in peak torque than under deception or nonfeedback training conditions.

SELECTION OF TEST PROTOCOL

Several factors influence ultimate selection of test protocol, including the muscle group to be tested, the stage of progression through a rehabilitation program, and the age and overall physical status of the patient or athlete. For example, surgical repair of a recurrent dislocating glenohumeral joint may preclude testing through an extreme of external rotation of the shoulder. As such, isokinetic exercise and assessment might occur through a restricted range of joint motion.

You should be careful, of course, when employing isokinetic exercise or assessment with patients who may be cardiovascularly compromised through age, risk factors, or inactivity. Both slow and high velocity isokinetic exercise of the trunk (Peel & Alland, 1990) and extremities (Douris, 1991) place significant demands on the cardiovascular system. Slow velocity isokinetic exercise may mimic isometric resistance in the sense that intrathoracic and intraabdominal pressure will be increased if the patient uses the Valsalva (breath holding) maneuver. Similarly, repeated slow or high speed isokinetic contractions of a major muscle group place considerable stress on the cardiovascular system. Maximal isokinetic resistance may be contraindicated in patients experiencing an unrelated compromise of the cardiorespiratory system. When any question exists, cardiovascular responses should be monitored during isokinetic exercise (Negus, Rippe, Freedson, & Michaels, 1987).

Frequent modifications in test protocol make intrasubject and intersubject comparisons difficult. For example, inconsistencies in lever-arm placement or damp setting may make an individual appear to be stronger or weaker during the retest when no change in strength has occurred. Moreover, inconsistency in number of warm-up and test repetitions, test velocities, and the isokinetic parameters evaluated renders comparison among a variety of athletic and nonathletic subjects within a clinical facility difficult. With that in mind, perhaps the best advice for clinicians and scientists is simply to be consistent in the selection of test protocols. Use of consistent protocols will permit creation of a bank of *normal* data that can be used to prescribe and monitor exercise protocols and aid in determining when a patient is prepared to assume activities of daily living or when an athlete is ready to resume strenuous activity.

This generic test protocol encompasses many of the essential components alluded to in the preceding paragraphs. Further considerations for isokinetic exercise and assessment are provided in Part II.

Recommended Protocol for Isokinetic Assessment of Human Muscle Performance

1. Musculoskeletal screening
2. General body stretching and warm-up
3. Patient setup with optimal stabilization
4. Alignment of joint and dynamometer axes of rotation
5. Verbal introduction to isokinetic concept of exercise
6. Gravity correction when appropriate
7. Warm-up (3 submaximal, 3 maximal repetitions)
8. Rest (30 s to 1 min)
9. Maximal test at slow velocity (4 to 6 repetitions)
10. Rest (30 s to 1 min)
11. Maximal test at fast velocity (4 to 6 repetitions)
12. Rest (30 s to 1 min)
13. Multiple repetition endurance test
14. Testing of contralateral extremity
15. Recording of test details to insure replication on retest
16. Explanation of results to patient

EFFECTS OF ISOKINETIC EXERCISE

Isokinetic exercise is a desirable form of resistance for rehabilitation for reasons mentioned in the introduction. However, isokinetic dynamometry is usually only one of several therapeutic interventions used during the rehabilitation of significant musculoskeletal injuries. For example, continuous passive motion, isometric and isotonic resistance, and functional activities of daily living or athletic participation may all have an important place in the rehabilitation process. Nevertheless, the effects of isokinetic exercise on muscle performance are well documented.

It is clear that maximal-effort concentric isokinetic training increases concentric peak torque, work, and power (Costill, Coyle, Fink, Lesmes, & Witzmann, 1979; Coyle et al., 1981; Lesmes, Costill, Coyle, & Fink, 1978; Perrin, Lephart, & Weltman, 1989). The mechanism for the increases in strength resulting from isokinetic training appears to be related to enhancement of glycolytic, ATP-CP, and Krebs cycle enzymatic activities (Costill et al., 1979), the ability to recruit more motor units, and perhaps recruitment of motor units in a more economical fashion (Coyle et al., 1981). Interestingly, the increases in strength resulting from isokinetic training frequently occur in the absence of increases in muscle cross-sectional girth and hypertrophy (Lesmes et al., 1978). This point would seem to further support the enzymatic and neural mechanisms mentioned previously. It has been postulated that the failure of isokinetic resistance to produce substantial muscle hypertrophy may have been due to the absence of an eccentric mode of contraction during training on prototype isokinetic dynamometry (Cote et al., 1988). Further research is needed to examine the effect of eccentric isokinetic exercise with active dynamometry on the cross-sectional size of muscle.

The specificity of concentric and eccentric training on strength acquisition is controversial. Specificity of training would suggest that concentric training produces increases in concentric strength and eccentric training produces increases in eccentric strength. But some research (Tomberlin et al., 1991) supports this theory, while other research refutes it (Petersen et al., 1990). One study of rotator cuff strengthening found concentric training increased concentric and eccentric strength and that eccentric training increased concentric but not eccentric strength (Ellenbecker, Davies, & Rowinski, 1988). These inconsistencies suggest that more research is needed.

VELOCITY SPECTRUM EXERCISE

Rehabilitation protocols frequently use exercise over a range of angular velocities, which has been termed *velocity spectrum* exercise. Clinicians who use velocity spectrum exercise protocols empirically report desirable results, although the physiological rationale for these protocols is somewhat unclear. Two possible explanations exist that are based on differential muscle fibers and recruitment patterns in mammalian skeletal muscles.

In general, human muscle fibers are classified as either Type I (slow twitch, ST) or Type II (fast twitch, FT), with varying subclassifications of the FT fiber (Brooke & Kaiser, 1970; Guth & Samaha, 1969; Peter, Barnard, Edgerton, Gillespie, & Stempel, 1972). ST fibers have motor units that are activated at lower thresholds and have low conduction velocities and long twitch contraction times. The ST fibers are specialized for protracted usage at relatively low velocities. FT fibers, on the other hand, have high threshold motor units with high conduction velocities and short twitch contraction times. The FT fibers are specialized for high power outputs and high velocities for short periods of time (Green, 1986). The recruitment of the respective fiber types depends on the tension requirements of a given muscular contraction. Because ST fibers have a low threshold for activation, they are recruited first. FT fibers are then recruited as more tension is required for movement (Sherman et al., 1982).

On one hand, based on these physiological characteristics, it would seem logical that slow velocity isokinetic exercise would recruit primarily ST fibers, and high velocity exercise would recruit primarily FT fibers. On the other hand, the maximal force output required during isokinetic contraction would be expected to require maximal or near maximal recruitment of both ST and FT fibers, independent of angular velocity. The literature seems to support the recruitment of both fibers rather than selective recruitment of ST and FT fibers based on exercise velocity. Any value of velocity spectrum exercise is more likely related to variations in the order of motor unit recruitment than to the recruitment of one fiber type in the absence of activation of another type.

STRENGTH OVERFLOW

A great deal of attention has been given to the overflow of increases in concentric isokinetic strength from an exercised velocity to both slower and faster velocities. In general, the literature seems to indicate that high velocity training is not as "specific" as slow exercise training. Training at fast velocities tends to increase strength at and below the exercise velocity. In contrast, exercise at slow velocities tends to produce increases specific to (or only slightly above) the training velocity (Coyle et al., 1981; Lesmes et al., 1978). The clinical relevance of this phenomenon is that patients who are unable to tolerate the higher levels of tension associated with slow isokinetic exercise may benefit from training at exclusively high velocities.

More recent evidence suggests that eccentric training does not have the same velocity specificity and overflow characteristics seen with concentric exercise. It appears that eccentric training at one speed tends to increase strength at both slower and faster test velocities (Duncan, Chandler, Cavanaugh, Johnson, & Buehler, 1989; Ryan, Magidow, & Duncan, 1991). Further research is needed to confirm this observation.

SELECTION OF EXERCISE PROTOCOL

When selecting an isokinetic exercise protocol consider such factors as duration and velocity of exercise, the range of joint motion through which the exercise is performed, and the length-tension relationship of the muscle group to be exercised. Each of these components will be dictated by the nature of the injury to the musculoskeletal system. I will present general guidelines for selection of test protocol here; details of specific injuries and body regions will be discussed in Part II.

Duration of Exercise

Costill et al. (1979) compared 6 and 30 seconds of isokinetic knee extension exercise and reported that substantial increases in muscle lactate occurred only from the 30-second bout of exercise. Indeed, even when the amount of total work during 30-second bouts of exercise was equated by use of repeated 6-second exercise bouts, only one of several markers of glycolytic, ATP-CP, and Krebs cycle enzyme activity increased. As such, the stimulus responsible for increasing muscle enzyme activities is more related to duration of a single bout of exercise than to the total work performed over several shorter bouts of exercise (Costill et al., 1979). These observations seem to support the use of isokinetic exercise protocols that will elevate the enzymatic activities associated with glycolytic, ATP-PC, and Krebs cycle metabolism. Moreover, the duration of isokinetic exercise should be based on the element of time rather than on the number of repetitions. Because isokinetic exercise is performed at a predetermined and fixed velocity, low speeds through a given range of motion will take more time than high speeds (Rothstein, Delitto, Sinacore, & Rose, 1983). For example, 30 repetitions at 90 deg/s through a 90 deg arc of motion would take 30 seconds, while 30 repetitions at 180 deg/s through the same range of motion would take only 15 seconds. A period of 30 seconds of exercise is recommended regardless of angular velocity.

Recommended Isokinetic Exercise Protocol

1. Musculoskeletal screening
2. General body stretching and warm-up
3. Patient setup for optimal stabilization and muscle length-tension relationship that replicates patient activities
4. Alignment of joint and dynamometer axes of rotation
5. Submaximal warm-up for familiarization with exercise velocity
6. Exercise at slow velocity (30-s duration)
7. Rest
8. Warm-up and exercise at intermediate velocity (30-s duration)
9. Rest
10. Warm-up and exercise at fast velocity (30-s duration)
11. Repeated exercise bouts at different muscle length-tension positions
12. General body stretching and cool-down
13. Ice application to involved joint or muscle group (20 min)

Note. The isokinetic exercise protocol should include concentric and eccentric contractions. If an eccentric mode is unavailable, contemporary isotonic equipment or free weights should be used to assure inclusion of eccentric contraction in the exercise program.

Range of Motion and Length-Tension Relationships

Whenever possible, exercise should occur through a complete range of joint motion to optimize the contraction-coupling process of actin and myosin within the muscle's sarcomeres. However, pathology within a joint occasionally precludes the use of isokinetic exercise through certain parts of the available range of motion. For example, patellofemoral joint forces during isokinetic knee extension exercise are 5.1 times greater than body weight at large angles (60-80 deg) of knee joint flexion, yet are dramatically reduced at low (0-30 deg) flexion angles (Kaufman, Kai-Nan, Litchy, Morrey, & Chao, 1991). The obvious clinical implication is that patients experiencing patellofemoral pain should perform isokinetic exercise through a range of motion restricted to low flexion angles.

Give the length-tension relationship of the exercised muscle group special attention when designing an isokinetic exercise protocol. While there may be value to varying the length-tension relationship of the target muscle group, exercise should occur primarily from a position that mimics the patient's activities of daily living or athletic activity. For example, it would seem illogical to restrict exercise of the rotator cuff in a pitcher to a position of complete shoulder adduction. Exercise from a 90 deg abducted position more closely approximates the position of the shoulder during the throwing motion (see Figure 3.17, a and b). Similarly, exercise of the thigh musculature exclusively from the seated position does not approximate the position of the hip during running; it can be better approximated by exercise from the prone or supine position (see Figure 3.18, a and b). I will

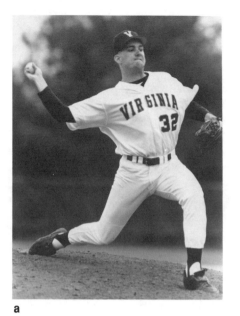
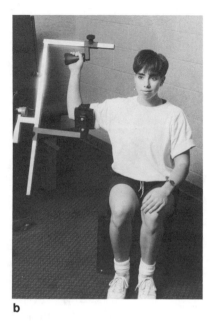

a   b

Figure 3.17   Isokinetic test and exercise position of the shoulder internal and external rotator muscles designed to replicate the position of the shoulder during the throwing motion. (Photo [a] by David Greene.)

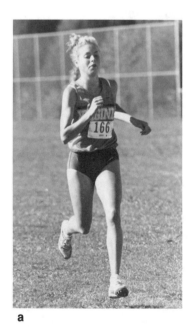
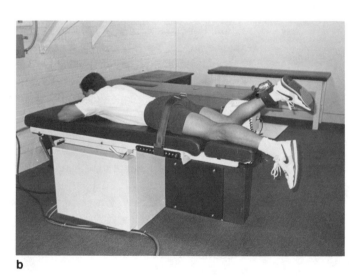

a   b

Figure 3.18   Isokinetic test and exercise position of the quadriceps and hamstring muscles designed to replicate the length-tension relationship during running. (Photos by David Green [a] and Teddy Worrell [b].)

present examples of modified joint positions for each joint in Part II. Then I'll leave it to you to match the joint position that approximates the length-tension relationship of the muscle group, patient, and activity in question.

Submaximal Isokinetic Exercise

The primary benefit of isokinetic resistance is that maximal overload of a muscle group can be achieved throughout a joint's available range of motion. In cases where maximal contraction may not be appropriate, isokinetic exercise may also be used to provide a submaximal form of resistance. For example, injury to the neuromuscular or articular systems may render a maximal contraction either impossible or inappropriate, so a percentage of the uninvolved side's peak torque may be used for submaximal exercise of the injured extremity. Instantaneous feedback from a numerical, digital, audio, or visual display may be useful in helping a patient perform at a predetermined submaximal level of exercise.

Chapter 4

Interpreting an Isokinetic Evaluation

The profile obtained from an isokinetic evaluation may be used to predict susceptibility to injury in a healthy individual, to monitor an injured patient's rehabilitation, or to determine readiness to return to activities of daily living or athletic participation after a therapeutic exercise program. Depending on instrument capabilities, interpreting an isokinetic evaluation usually involves careful analysis of the subject's ability to generate torque, work, or power.

MEASURING PEAK TORQUE, WORK, AND POWER

Torque may be assessed as either a peak or an average value. Peak torque is often obtained from the highest point of one of several isokinetic torque curves. However, because several isokinetic contractions are necessary to obtain a true peak value, the average of the peak points from several consecutive torque curves (average peak torque) may be a better indicator of the maximum performance of a given muscle group. The primary advantage of using peak values of torque is that muscle performance can be assessed where full range of joint motion may be restricted.

Average torque is measured from the complete tracing of one or several consecutive isokinetic curves. The primary advantage of this value is that artifacts that might occur in the torque curve from deceleration of the limb and lever arm have a less dramatic effect than on a measure of peak torque or force. Because this measure is obtained from the complete isokinetic curve, however, you must ensure that the range of motion tested is consistent, both between injured and uninjured sides and within the injured side in subsequent evaluations throughout a rehabilitation program. As I noted in chapter 1, where complete range of motion exists, the relationship between peak and average values for both torque and force is quite high. So any of these measures is likely to provide adequate information on the performance of a given muscle group, assuming adherence to consistent test protocols.

The work capacity of a single muscle group may be determined by calculating the total area under one or a series of consecutive torque curves. Power is determined by assessing the time required to perform work within a single or several repetitions. Some isokinetic instrumentation has computer software capable of reporting each of these parameters.

MEASURING ENDURANCE

Endurance is the capacity of a muscle to produce force over a series of consecutive isokinetic contractions. Isokinetic endurance is often quantified by the number of repetitions required for the maximum torque value in a repetition to fall below 50% of the maximum value recorded in the first repetition (Figure 4.1) or by the percent decline over a certain number of repetitions or amount of time. Endurance has also been expressed as a fatigue index. For example, Thorstensson and Karlsson (1976) defined endurance as the torque from the last three contractions as a percentage of the initial three contractions of 50 contractions. However, Kannus, Cook, and Alosa (1992) reported that a fatigue index as a measure of endurance was less repeatable and gave misleading information about the effect of training on endurance. I have also questioned the reliability of this procedure (Perrin, 1986).

Because computer interfacing with isokinetic dynamometers now enables quantification of work, the total work performed over several isokinetic

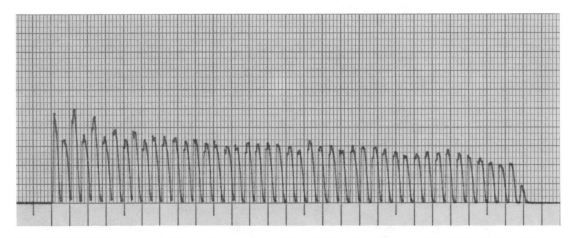

Figure 4.1   Repeated contractions of an agonist and antagonist muscle group to assess endurance. The number of contractions from the initial peak torque to 50% of the initial peak is noted as the endurance factor. The first, third, fifth, etc., curves are quadriceps contractions and the second, fourth, sixth, etc., curves are hamstring contractions. Note how the quadriceps decrease more rapidly than do the hamstrings over the course of this endurance test. Since this test occurred from the seated position, this observation may be related to the quadriceps contracting against the effect of gravity while the hamstrings are assisted by gravity.

contractions may be a better indicator of the endurance capacity of a single muscle group. Indeed, Kannus et al. (1992) reported that the work performed during the last 5 of 25 repetitions and the total work performed were as valuable and consistent as peak torque measurements. Also, these measures were valuable in documentation of progress during endurance training.

FORCE-VELOCITY RELATIONSHIPS

Isokinetic dynamometers enable assessment and exercise throughout a range of velocities. Depending on instrumentation, this potential velocity spectrum may range from 1 to 500 deg/s. Accurate interpretation of an isokinetic evaluation requires an understanding of the force-velocity relationship during both concentric and eccentric contraction.

The ability of a muscle to generate concentric force is greatest at slow isokinetic velocities and decreases linearly as the test velocity increases. Figure 4.2 illustrates decreases in concentric peak torque when isokinetic test velocity increases from 60 to 240 deg/s. Recognition of this phenomenon is paramount to accurate interpretation of normal single muscle group strength and reciprocal muscle group relationships.

The force-velocity curve produced during eccentric exercise is quite different from the curve resulting from concentric muscular contraction. For ex-

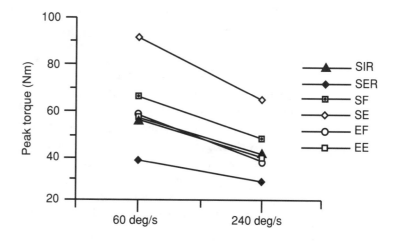

Figure 4.2   Peak torque of the shoulder internal (SIR) and external (SER) rotator, shoulder flexor (SF) and extensor (SE), and elbow flexor (EF) and extensor (EE) muscle groups at a slow and fast speed of contraction. A decrease in peak torque with increase in test velocity is seen for all muscle groups tested.

Data from "Relationship Between Shoulder and Elbow Isokinetic Peak Torque, Torque Acceleration Energy, Average Power, and Total Work and Throwing Velocity in Intercollegiate Pitchers" by D. Pawlowski and D.H. Perrin, 1989, *Athletic Training, 24*, pp. 129-132.

ample, while concentric force decreases with increases in test velocity, eccentric force remains the same, and sometimes even increases in force production. The physiological mechanism for the discrepancy in the concentric and eccentric force-velocity relationship appears to be related to differences in the binding and interaction of actin and myosin within the muscle sarcomere (see the illustration on p. 72, also see Stauber, 1989a). Upon activation of the excitation-contraction coupling mechanism, myosin binds to actin as inhibitory factors on the actin binding site are removed by the release of calcium. Once attachment has occurred, the potential energy stored in the myosin filament is transformed into the mechanical events of the cross-bridge action. This produces tension, or concentric shortening of the muscle. If the external resistance exceeds the cross-bridge ability to shorten (eccentric contraction), the actin-myosin bond is broken before transduction of energy can occur. As the external force continues, the energized myosin is repeatedly reattached and pulled apart from the actin without transduction of energy. Not only does this process produce greater tension at a given sarcomere length than does shortening (concentric) contraction, it is also independent of velocity until the velocity of lengthening exceeds the binding rate of the actin and myosin. The practical application is that as velocity of concentric contraction increases, fewer cross bridges are formed and thus less force is produced. In contrast, the cross bridge is not required to undergo the complete series of chemical events during eccentric contraction, and so the ability to generate tension at higher test velocities is not adversely affected. The data in Figure 4.3 help explain the concentric and eccentric force-velocity relationship. Note that at a test velocity of 60 deg/s, eccentric peak torque is greater than concentric peak torque. Also, as test velocity increases to 180 deg/s, concentric peak torque decreases while eccentric peak torque actually increases. These clinical observations are consistent with the physiological explanation discussed by Stauber (1989a).

Considerable research has examined both the isometric and isotonic force curves. Human muscle was thought to have the greatest potential to produce force via an isometric (zero velocity) contraction, until the advent of eccentric isokinetic dynamometry disproved this theory. Less concentric isotonic force is produced than isometric force at a slow velocity of contraction. As test velocity increases, isotonic force decreases linearly and produces a hyperbolic force-velocity curve. Little controversy now exists in the literature with regard to these points.

The eccentric force-velocity curve has been thoroughly described in animal studies using in vitro isolated muscle preparations. Only recently has isokinetic dynamometry been developed that offers the ability to assess in vivo eccentric contraction of human muscle. Recent studies have demonstrated that the eccentric force-velocity curve for intact human muscle is somewhat different than for isolated animal muscle. In general, lengthening contraction

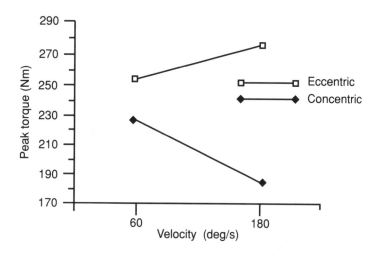

Figure 4.3   Concentric and eccentric peak torque of the hamstring muscle group at two test velocities. Note that concentric peak torque decreases with an increase in test velocity and for this muscle group, eccentric peak torque increases with an increase in test velocity.

Data from "Comparison of Isokinetic Strength and Flexibility Measures Between Hamstring Injured and Noninjured Athletes" by T.W. Worrell, D.H. Perrin, B.M. Gansneder, and J.H. Gieck, 1991, *Journal of Orthopaedic and Sports Physical Therapy*, **13**, pp. 118-125.

of isolated animal muscle exceeds isometric levels and increases substantially with increases in test velocity (Hill, 1938) (Figure 4.4). Eccentric contraction in intact human muscle also exceeds isometric levels, but often increases only slightly with increases in test velocity (Westing, Seger, Karlson, & Ekblom, 1988) (Figure 4.5). The mechanism for this difference in isolated animal muscle and human muscle has been postulated to be related to a neural inhibitory system in humans. Some have suggested that this neural safety mechanism results from inhibitory feedback from Golgi tendon organs, cutaneous, pain, and joint receptors, and free nerve endings within muscle (Westing, Cresswell, & Thorstensson, 1991). That is, as eccentric force exceeds isometric levels, the inhibitory system is subconsciously engaged to protect the human muscle from injury. Interestingly, electrical stimulation superimposed on maximal volitional eccentric, isometric, and isotonic contractions increases eccentric force by as much as 25%, but has no enhancing effect on either isometric or isotonic contractions (Westing, Seger, & Thorstensson, 1990). This observation seems to support the theory of a neural inhibiting system.

Reviews of the eccentric force-velocity curve in humans have revealed some inconsistencies. These inconsistencies are probably related to differences between selected muscle groups (Westing et al., 1988), between men and women (Colliander & Tesch, 1989), and between low- and high-trained

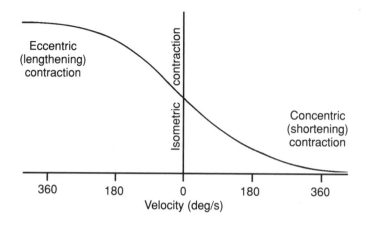

Figure 4.4   Concentric and eccentric force-velocity curve resulting from in vitro isolated animal muscle.

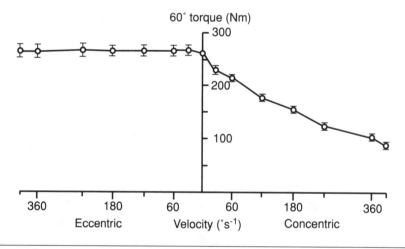

Figure 4.5   Mean (± standard error of mean) 60 deg angle-specific knee extensor torque output under maximal voluntary eccentric and concentric constant-velocity loading at 30, 60, 120, 180, 270, 360, and 400 deg/s, plus an isometric test at 60 deg of knee angle (males, n=21).

Data from "Eccentric and Concentric Torque-Velocity Characteristics of the Quadriceps Femoris in Man" by S.H. Westing, J.Y. Seger, E. Karlson, and B. Ekblom, 1988, *European Journal of Applied Physiology, 58*, pp. 100-104.

individuals (Hortobagyi & Katch, 1990). For example, Colliander and Tesch (1989) reported that eccentric peak torque did not increase with increasing test velocity in males but did increase in females. Hortobagyi and Katch (1990) grouped subjects according to either high strength (HS) or low strength (LS). They found that with increases in test velocity, eccentric torque increased in the HS subjects but did not increase in the LS subjects. These differences were hypothesized to be related to a decreased or absent neural inhibitory mechanism in the trained subjects.

So, the eccentric force-velocity curve in human muscle appears to remain essentially constant or increase only slightly with increases in test velocity. Figure 4.6 illustrates the normal concentric, and eccentric torque-velocity characteristics in a group of female subjects. Studies that show a decrease in eccentric torque at high test velocities may not be assessing eccentric torque though a range of motion great enough to generate maximum volitional eccentric force (Griffin, 1987). In any event, the development and refinement of active isokinetic dynamometry creates an exciting new area for research into eccentric human muscle performance.

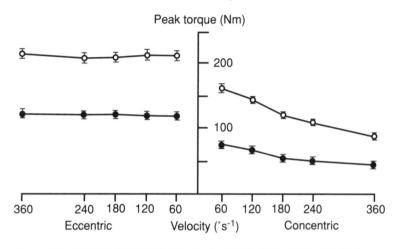

Figure 4.6   Mean (± standard error of mean) maximal voluntary knee extensor (open symbols) and knee flexor (closed symbols) torque output (peak values corrected for gravitational effects) under eccentric and concentric constant-velocity loading at 60, 120, 180, 240, and 360 deg/s (females, *n*=20).

Data from "Eccentric and Concentric Torque-Velocity Characteristics, Torque Output Comparisons, and Gravity Effect Torque Corrections for the Quadriceps and Hamstring Muscles in Females" by S.H. Westing and J.Y. Seger, 1989, *International Journal of Sports Medicine*, **10**, pp. 175-180.

PEAK TORQUE RELATIVE TO BODY WEIGHT

A plethora of data have been reported on normal absolute strength values for several muscle groups in a variety of athletic and sedentary populations. This information serves as a basis for determining adequate levels of peak torque in these populations. However, the variations in body size and somatotype within both athletic and sedentary groups presents a challenge in determining an adequate level of torque for all individuals. One technique that is useful in individualizing the interpretation of an isokinetic evaluation is to express torque or force relative to total body weight. For example, one study encountered difficulty when attempting to compare strength between football, lacrosse, and track athletes because of substantial differences in body size among these subjects (Worrell, Perrin, Gansneder, & Gieck, 1991). To account for these differences, peak torque values of the quadriceps and hamstring muscle groups were divided by each subject's body weight, yielding a Newton meter per kilogram (Nm/kg) value. Peak torque expressed relative to total body weight enabled comparisons to be made between these subjects in spite of the marked discrepancies in body size. Some isokinetic instrumentation automatically expresses peak torque or force values as a percentage of body weight for each muscle group assessed. This practice is especially common when expressing normal strength values for muscles acting on the knee and trunk.

Isokinetic strength may also be expressed as a percentage of lean body mass. The difference in strength between males and females is reduced when expressed relative to total body weight, and these differences are reduced even further when expressed relative to lean body mass. Unfortunately, humans cannot shed their adipose tissue when performing activities of daily living or participating in athletics. Thus, even though a high correlation has been reported between these two ways of expressing strength (Smith, Mayer, Gatchel, & Becker, 1985), it is probably more appropriate to express strength as a percentage of total body weight rather than lean body mass.

I advise caution when you are interpreting strength values expressed relative to body weight. Peak torque expressed as Nm of torque/lb of body weight yields a very different number than when expressed as Nm of torque/kg of body weight. For example, if a 150-lb individual produced 125 ft-lb of torque with the quadriceps muscle group, the torque to body weight ratio (125 ft-lb/150 lb) would be .83. If this same relationship was expressed in SI units (170 Nm/68 kg) the ratio would be 2.5. Interpretation of this relationship would be confounded even further if incorrectly expressed as Nm of torque/lb of body weight. This calculation (170 Nm/150 lb) would yield a ratio of 1.13. Unfortunately, many reports of strength relative to body weight in the literature do not describe exactly how values were derived. Clinicians and researchers should succinctly state the units of measure used to express strength relative to body weight. If all data were expressed in accordance with SI units (Nm/kg), meaningful comparisons could be made across studies through use of meta-analysis.

BILATERAL MUSCLE GROUP COMPARISONS

A distinct advantage with assessment of single muscle groups of the extremities is that normally a contralateral muscle group may be assessed as a basis for comparison. Should bilateral comparisons be made, it is obviously essential that the test protocol for right and left sides be consistent in all respects. For example, the injured side may be restricted to some degree in the range of motion available for isokinetic assessment. Even though complete motion is likely available in the uninjured extremity, the range of motion to be tested should be identical to the injured side. Testing through bilaterally unequal ranges of motion could confound interpretation of the isokinetic report for several reasons. Greater prestretch to a muscle may enable that muscle to produce a higher level of peak torque within the subsequent range of motion tested. Comparisons in average torque would also be confounded because the average value is determined from each point along the isokinetic curve. Comparison of work values (total area under the torque curve) would also be invalid because a greater range of motion would permit greater amounts of total work.

Variations in placement of the lever arm's resistance pad between right and left sides could also confound the bilateral comparisons of peak or average torque. Moreover, should a dual pad resistance device (see chapter 6) be used on an anterior cruciate ligament–deficient or reconstructed knee, it should also be used for assessment of the uninjured side. Because torque is force produced by a muscle about a joint's axis of rotation, variations or modifications in placement of one or more resistance pads may affect production of peak or average torque.

Many clinicians assume that torque values for the uninjured extremity can be used as the standard for return of the injured extremity to a normal state during rehabilitation. Confounding this interpretation is the influence of limb dominance, or in the case of athletes, the effect of neuromuscular specificity of various sport activities on bilateral strength relationships. In general, few bilateral differences are found in the lower extremities of sedentary individuals and most athletes. Athletes in bilaterally symmetrical upper extremity sport activities (e.g., swimming) have few differences between dominant and nondominant sides. However, athletes in bilaterally asymmetrical upper extremity activities (e.g., throwing) may have dominant side muscle group strength as much as 15% greater than the nondominant side (Perrin, Robertson, & Ray, 1987). Figure 4.7, a-c illustrates bilateral comparisons of shoulder internal rotation peak torque, work, and power in nonathletes, swimmers, and pitchers. Clinicians, then, must consider the industrial or athletic activities of their patients when assessing upper extremity muscle groups. For example, rehabilitation of the internal rotator muscle group of a competitive pitcher to the strength level of the uninjured nondominant side is probably inadequate in preparation for a return to pitching. Chapters 5 and 6 present normative bilateral strength data for the upper and lower extremities in a variety of sedentary and athletic populations.

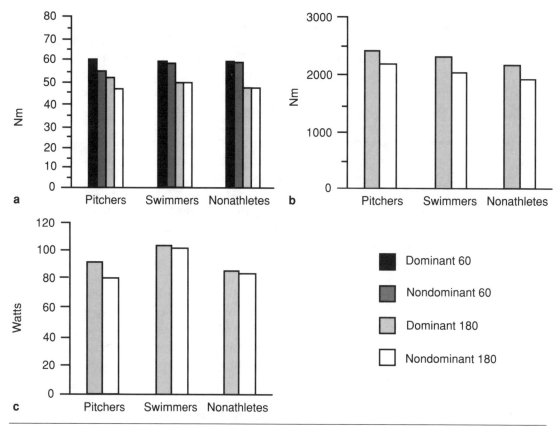

Figure 4.7　Shoulder internal rotation peak torque at 60 and 180 deg/s (a), work at 180 deg/s (b), and power at 180 deg/s (c) of the dominant and nondominant sides. Note the asymmetry between dominant and nondominant side values in pitchers compared to swimmers and nonathletes, particularly with respect to peak torque (a) and power (c).

Data from "Bilateral Isokinetic Peak Torque, Torque Acceleration Energy, Power, and Work Relationships in Athletes and Nonathletes" by D.H. Perrin, R.J. Robertson, and R.L. Ray, 1987, *Journal of Orthopaedic and Sports Physical Therapy, 9*, pp. 184-189.

RECIPROCAL MUSCLE GROUP COMPARISONS

The muscle groups on both sides of a joint necessarily act reciprocally to produce smooth and coordinated motion. When a muscle group produces a desired joint action it is the agonist for the observed motion. The muscle group producing the opposite joint action is the antagonist. For example, to produce extension of the knee joint, the quadriceps contracts in a concentric fashion, acting as the agonist for the observed joint action. In knee extension, the hamstring muscle group relaxes by the principle of reciprocal inhibition; it is the antagonist for the observed action. Conversely, to produce knee flexion, the hamstring muscle group contracts in a concentric fashion (agonist), and the quadriceps muscle group relaxes (antagonist) during the observed action. The respective roles of the quadriceps and hamstring muscle groups in producing extension and flexion of the knee joint also require that the antagonist act in an eccentric fashion to decelerate the limb near the conclusion of the observed joint action. For example, during the final phase of knee extension, the hamstring muscle group contracts in an eccentric (lengthening) manner to terminate the observed motion. During flexion of the knee, the quadriceps muscle group contracts in an eccentric manner to terminate flexion of the knee. The strength relationship of these two muscle groups is known as the reciprocal muscle group ratio.

Strength training specialists have long recognized the importance of training both of the muscle groups producing opposite actions about a joint (e.g., flexors and extensors, abductors and adductors, internal and external rotators). In spite of this attention to training, one muscle group usually tends to be stronger than the other. It has been postulated (though not scientifically proven) that excessive imbalances in reciprocal muscle group ratios predispose the joint or weaker muscle group to injury. Because of this, the ratios about most major joints have received considerable attention in preseason screening and rehabilitation of athletes.

Determination of a "normal" reciprocal muscle group ratio may be confounded by several factors. As previously noted, failure to gravity correct during isokinetic assessment may artificially inflate or deflate the strength of one muscle group relative to another. Test velocity may also dramatically influence the determination of reciprocal muscle group ratios, particularly during concentric isokinetic assessment. Using the thigh musculature as an example, quadriceps torque will decrease more than hamstring torque with increases in test velocity (Fillyaw et al., 1986). This means that a lower hamstring/quadriceps reciprocal muscle group ratio will be found at slower test velocities, yet the hamstring muscle group will appear to be stronger relative to the quadriceps muscle group as test velocity increases. It should be noted that gravity correction procedures help to adjust for this error when determining the hamstring/quadriceps ratio throughout a velocity spectrum of testing (Appen & Duncan, 1986; Fillyaw et al., 1986).

It is interesting that virtually all studies of upper and lower extremity reciprocal muscle group ratios report concentric to concentric or eccentric to eccentric ratios. For example, the concentric hamstring to concentric quadriceps muscle group ratios are typically reported, and the same is usually found for the shoulder external to internal rotator ratios. However, the hamstring muscle group's eccentric contraction is essential for deceleration of knee extension during sprinting, as is the shoulder external rotator's eccentric contraction during deceleration of shoulder internal rotation during throwing. This kinesiological observation would seem to support reporting of quadriceps concentric to hamstring eccentric ratios, and shoulder concentric internal rotator to eccentric external rotator reciprocal muscle group ratios. Perhaps the advent of active isokinetic dynamometry will bring more reports of these concentric to eccentric ratios to the scientific literature.

RETURN TO ACTIVITY

The capacity of human muscle to perform may be compromised by any of several factors. Injury to any component of the muscle-tendon unit (e.g., strain, rupture, tendinitis) will limit that muscle's ability to produce force. Injury to a joint frequently results in alienation of the involved body part (e.g., limping, immobilization), which can very quickly result in marked atrophy of the muscles acting on that joint. Muscle may also atrophy if it receives inadequate innervation from the nervous system. Isokinetic assessment is particularly useful in determining when a muscle group has been adequately rehabilitated from any of these pathologic states and when it is prepared for safe return to physical activity.

Underscoring the value of an isokinetic evaluation, however, is the need to evaluate all components involved with rehabilitation of injury to the musculoskeletal system. In particular, strength, flexibility, proprioception, functional ability, and psychological status are all essential to returning to one's occupation or athletic endeavor. The following studies illustrate the fallacy of assessing only strength as the criterion to return to activity.

The first study examined the relationship between quadriceps and hamstring strength, flexibility, and knee joint displacement and functional capacity in a group of subjects who had sustained injury to the anterior cruciate ligament (Lephart, Perrin, Fu, Gieck, McCue, & Irrgang, 1992). The subjects were divided into two groups: those able to return and those unable to return to preinjury levels of physical activity following conservative (nonsurgical) management of the anterior cruciate ligament–deficient knee. The group unable to return had significant deficits in performance during a battery of controlled functional performance tests (Figure 4.8). Moreover, a stronger relationship was found between functional capacity and return to activity than between isokinetic strength and return to activity.

The second study compared strength and flexibility measures in the hamstring muscle group of injured and noninjured athletes matched by sport and position (Worrell et al., 1991). Isokinetic evaluation included assessing hamstring and quadriceps concentric and eccentric strength and reciprocal muscle group ratios. The group with a history of injury had significant deficits in flexibility of the hamstring muscle group compared to the uninjured side and to the uninjured group (Figure 4.9). However, no significant deficits in any isokinetic parameter were found in either extremity of either group. In particular, the hamstring/quadriceps reciprocal muscle group ratio at 60 deg/s was .61 for the hamstring injured extremity and .64 for the uninjured group's matched extremity.

The third study compared the relationship among isokinetic concentric and eccentric quadriceps and hamstring forces and three components of athletic performance in male athletes from five different sports (Anderson, Gieck, Perrin, Weltman, Rutt, & Denegar, 1991). The functional performance tests included a vertical jump, a 40-yard dash, and an agility run test. The study found little relationship between quadriceps or hamstring force and performance on the tests.

Restoring a muscle group to its preinjury level of performance is paramount during a rehabilitation program. However, as the previous studies illustrate, isokinetic evaluation is only one of several physiological factors that deserve consideration before successful return to activity can be achieved.

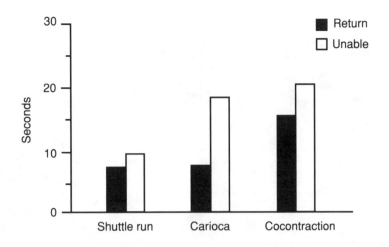

Figure 4.8 Performance on three functional tests in ACL–insufficient subjects. Those able to return to preinjury levels of activity performed significantly better in each test than those unable to return to activity.

Data from "Relationship Between Selected Physical Characteristics and Functional Capacity in the Anterior Cruciate Ligament–Insufficient Athlete" by S.M. Lephart, D.H. Perrin, F.H. Fu, J.H. Gieck, F.C. McCue, and J.J. Irrgang, 1992, *Journal of Orthopaedic and Sports Physical Therapy*, **16**, pp. 174-181.

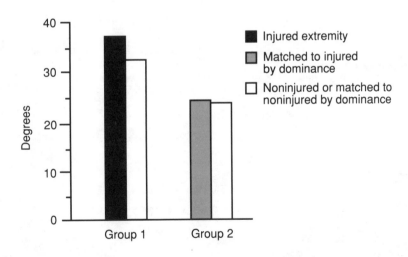

Figure 4.9 Hamstring flexibility values in degrees from full extension. Group 1 is hamstring injured subjects and Group 2 is nonhamstring injured subjects. Injured and noninjured extremities in Group 2 matched with Group 1 according to extremity dominance. Group 1 had significant deficits in flexibility in the absence of any deficits in strength or reciprocal muscle group ratios.

Data from "Comparison of Isokinetic Strength and Flexibility Measures Between Hamstring Injured and Noninjured Athletes" by T.W. Worrell, D.H. Perrin, B.M. Gansneder, and J.H. Gieck, 1991, *Journal of Orthopaedic and Sports Physical Therapy*, **13**, p. 123.

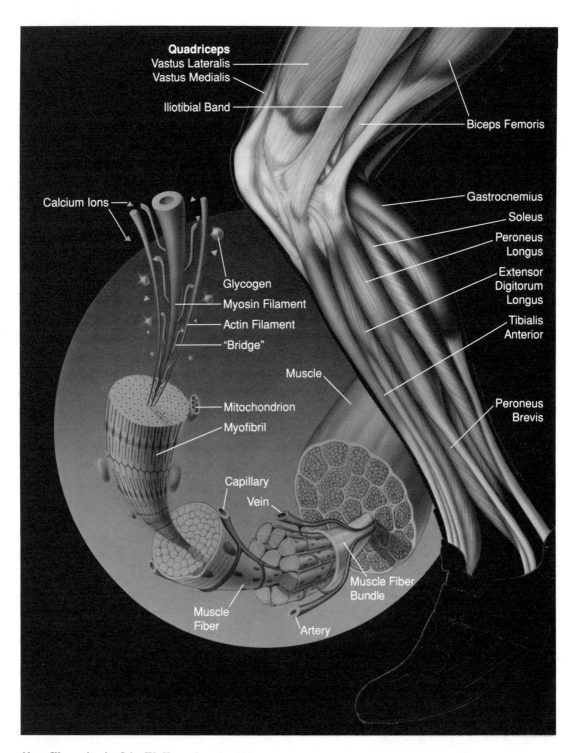

Quadriceps
Vastus Lateralis
Vastus Medialis

Iliotibial Band

Biceps Femoris

Gastrocnemius

Soleus

Peroneus
Longus

Extensor
Digitorum
Longus

Tibialis
Anterior

Peroneus
Brevis

Calcium Ions

Glycogen

Myosin Filament

Actin Filament

"Bridge"

Muscle

Mitochondrion

Myofibril

Capillary

Vein

Muscle Fiber
Bundle

Muscle
Fiber

Artery

Note. Illustration by John W. Karapelou, © 1992.

Part II

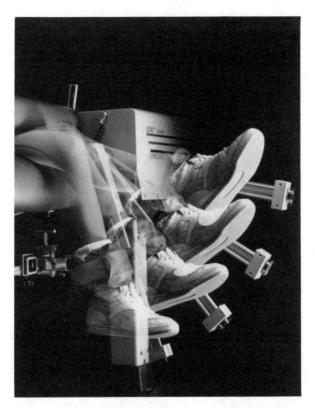

Clinical Application of Isokinetics

Part II addresses the kinesiology of each major joint of the upper and lower extremities and of the trunk. Guidelines for test positioning for optimum isolation of target muscle groups are presented. Isokinetic exercise through upper extremity functional patterns and lower extremity closed-kinetic-chain positions are also addressed. You will find the tables of normative data and reliability coefficients at the end of each chapter useful as guidelines for assessment of a variety of patient populations.

Chapter 5

Isokinetic Assessment and Exercise of the Upper Extremity

Clinicians and researchers are becoming increasingly interested in isokinetic exercise and assessment of the upper extremity. In this chapter, I discuss the muscles acting on the shoulder, elbow, forearm, and wrist and the use of isokinetic dynamometry for exercise through multiple-joint functional patterns. At the end of the chapter, you will find tables of normative data for each major muscle group of the upper extremity. The reliability of measuring upper extremity muscle performance is presented in the final table of the chapter.

THE SHOULDER JOINT

The shoulder joint consists of the articulation of the head of the humerus and the glenoid cavity of the scapula. The glenohumeral (g-h) joint is a complex multiaxial articulation capable of movement through each of the cardinal planes and through a variety of diagonal and horizontal patterns. Joint stability is provided primarily by capsular and muscular soft tissue structures rather than by the configuration of this rather shallow ball-and-socket articulation. Reliable assessment of the musculature of the region is especially difficult due to the multiple degrees of freedom and extensive mobility of the glenohumeral joint.

Shoulder Internal and External Rotation

Rotation of the glenohumeral joint through the transverse plane can be performed from the neutral position (adduction) (Figure 5.1), through the sagittal plane from the 90 deg abducted position (Figure 5.2, a and b), or anywhere in between. Shoulder rotation can also be performed through the coronal plane from a position of 90 deg of horizontal adduction (Figure 5.3). Internal rotation is produced by

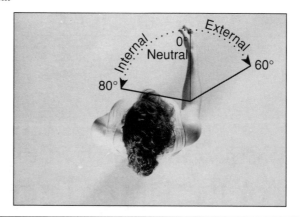

Figure 5.1   Shoulder internal and external rotation range of motion from the neutral (adducted) position.

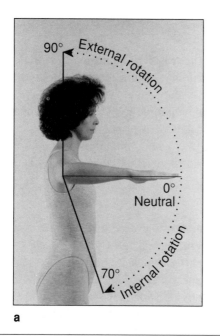

a

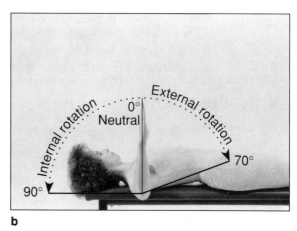

b

Figure 5.2   Shoulder internal and external rotation range of motion from the 90 deg abducted position in standing (a) and supine (b) positions.

the subscapularis, teres major, pectoralis major, latissimus dorsi, and anterior deltoid muscles, with the relative contribution from these muscles related to variations in their respective length-tension relationships as the glenohumeral joint moves from the neutral to 90 deg abducted position. External rotation is produced by the infraspinatus, teres minor, and posterior deltoid muscles.

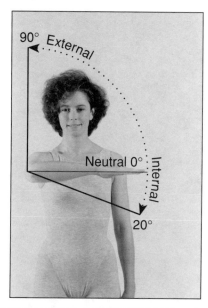

Figure 5.3 Shoulder internal and external rotation range of motion from 90 deg of horizontal adduction.

The tension required to produce a given rotational movement of the shoulder may also influence the relative contribution from the involved musculature. For example, EMG analysis of the shoulder musculature during the act of throwing indicates significant activity of the pectoralis major and latissimus dorsi muscles during the acceleration phase. In contrast, the subscapularis muscle remains relatively silent during this phase of throwing (Jobe, Radovich, Tibone, & Perry, 1984; Jobe, Tibone, Perry, & Moynes, 1983).

The optimal position for isokinetic exercise and assessment of shoulder rotation remains somewhat controversial. Some clinicians avoid exercise and assessment from the 90 deg abducted position for fear of inducing the symptoms associated with shoulder impingement syndrome. However, it is unlikely that the musculature involved in producing the forceful overhead internal rotation found in many athletic activities can be isolated from the neutral position. Logic dictates that if shoulder abduction is limited from surgical repair or the presence of impingement syndrome, exercise and assessment should be restricted to positions no greater than 45 deg of abduction. Otherwise, exercise should occur through a progression from the neutral to 90 deg abducted position (Figure 5.4, a-c). As with all joints, exercise and assessment should ultimately approximate as closely as possible the positional requirements of the shoulder for activities of daily living or athletic participation.

It has also been suggested that exercise and assessment of the shoulder rotator musculature should occur in the plane of the scapula (30 to 45

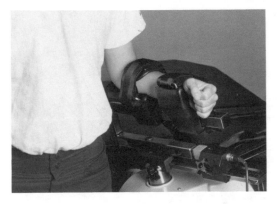

a

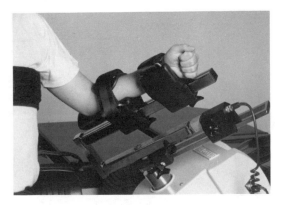

b

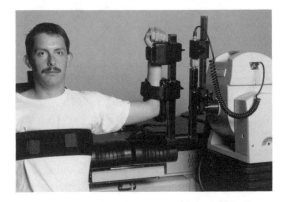

c

Figure 5.4   Test and exercise positions for the shoulder internal and external rotator muscles in a progression from neutral (a) to 45 deg (b) to 90 deg (c) of abduction.

deg anterior to the frontal plane) rather than the frontal plane (Greenfield, Donatelli, Wooden, & Wilkes, 1990; Hellwig & Perrin, 1991) (Figure 5.5, a and b). The basis of this recommendation is that most anatomists and clinicians describe motions of the shoulder relative to the trunk rather than to the scapula. Because movements of most distal bones are related to their proximal bones, reason suggests this should also be the case at the glenohumeral joint (Johnston, 1937). Moreover, clinicians also anecdotally report greater patient comfort when exercise or assessment occurs in the plane of the scapula. The effect of these two positions on torque production of the shoulder rotator musculature remains somewhat unclear and deserves further attention. For example, Greenfield et al. (1990) reported greater strength values for the external rotators in the plane of the scapula, whereas Hellwig and Perrin (1991) found no difference between positions for either the internal or external rotators.

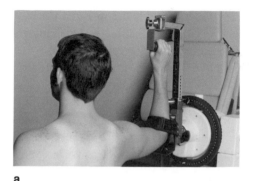 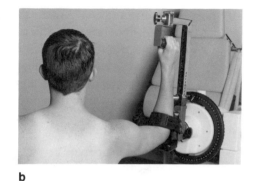

a   b

Figure 5.5   Isokinetic test and exercise positions for the shoulder internal and external rotator muscles in the frontal plane (a) and the plane of the scapula (b).

The variations in test position make interpretation of normative data for the shoulder rotator musculature somewhat complex. Table 5.1 presents normative values of shoulder internal and external rotation for a variety of populations and from test positions ranging from the neutral to 90 deg abducted positions. I advise you to carefully consider test position when making comparisons of shoulder rotation strength with values found in the scientific literature. In general, the external rotator muscles produce approximately 60% to 80% of the torque values generated by the internal rotator muscles (Table 5.2), and a comparison of the bilateral strength values of these muscle groups from Table 5.1 indicates a dominant/nondominant relationship usually within 10%. However, clinicians should consider the neuromuscular demands of a variety of athletic activities and their potential effect on the reciprocal and bilateral muscle group relationships of the shoulder rotator musculature. For example, a comparison of internal and external rotator muscle group strength values from normal subjects and the national water polo team (Table 5.2) revealed a ratio substantially lower in the athletic population (McMaster, Long, & Caiozzo, 1991). This would suggest a neuromuscular adaptation of the internal rotator muscle group relative to the external rotators in this particular population of athletes.

Failure to correct for the effect of gravity also confounds interpretation of normative data for the shoulder internal and external rotators. Few reports in the literature employed a gravity correction procedure when assessing shoulder rotation strength. However, the influence of gravity correction on assessment of this musculature has an effect similar to the quadriceps and hamstring muscle groups (Perrin et al., 1992). When assessed from a seated position, the absence of gravity correction significantly underpredicts the muscle group opposed by gravity (external rotators) and overpredicts the muscle group assisted by gravity (internal rotators). Although none of the studies in Table 5.2 reported the use of gravity correction, the procedure influences determination of the shoulder rotator reciprocal muscle group ratio. Because gravity correction adds to the external rotators and subtracts from the internal rotators, the external/internal rotation reciprocal muscle group ratio is appropriately higher, in some cases to the point where it approaches 1.0 (Perrin et al., 1992). These findings seem to support use of a gravity correction procedure for any muscle group tested within a gravity-dependent position. Clinicians should note the presence or absence of a gravity correction procedure when interpreting normative strength values of the shoulder musculature.

Shoulder Flexion and Extension

Flexion and extension of the glenohumeral joint occur through the sagittal plane (Figure 5.6, a and b). The muscles most involved in producing flexion include the anterior portion of the deltoid muscle and the clavicular portion of the pectoralis major muscle. Extension is produced by the sternal portion of the pectoralis major, the teres major, the posterior portion of the deltoid muscle, and most importantly by the powerful latissimus dorsi muscle. The biceps brachii and triceps muscles act as assistant movers during shoulder flexion and extension, respectively.

Figure 5.7, a and b illustrates two common positions for assessment and exercise of the shoulder flexor and extensor musculature. True isolation of

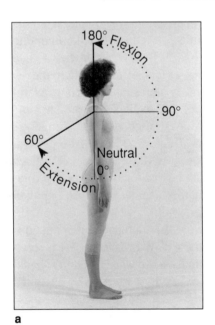
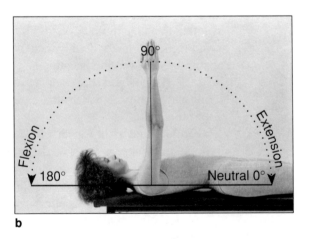

a   b

Figure 5.6   Shoulder flexion and extension ranges of motion in the standing (a) and supine (b) positions.

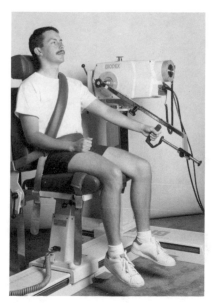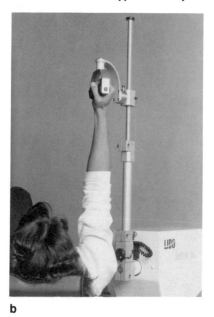

a   b

Figure 5.7   Test and exercise position for the shoulder flexor and extensor muscles while seated (a) and supine (b).

the shoulder flexors and extensors from this position is difficult because the elbow flexors and extensors must be prominently involved to maintain elbow extension during the assessment procedure. Moreover, maximal generation of shoulder flexion and extension depends on the ability of the subject to firmly grasp the handle of the lever arm. As such, you can accomplish better isolation of the shoulder flexor and extensor musculature by placing the resistance pad of the lever arm at the distal humerus, as shown in Figure 5.8. The contribution of the biceps brachii and triceps muscles can be minimized by maintaining elbow flexion during assessment of shoulder flexion and elbow extension during testing of the shoulder extensor musculature.

Normal isokinetic strength values for the shoulder flexor and extensor musculature may be found in Table 5.3. In nondisabled, nonathletic people or in athletes not requiring selected overuse of either the shoulder flexors or extensors, the shoulder flexor musculature has been shown to produce 75% to 85% of the torque values generated by the extensor muscles. However, some athletic activities require powerful extension of the shoulder joint (e.g., throwing, rowing, and swimming). This demand on the shoulder extensors tends to reduce the shoulder flexor/extensor reciprocal muscle group ratio to the point where the flexor muscles may produce only 50% of the torque values generated by the extensor muscles. For normal reciprocal muscle group ratios for a variety of populations, see Table 5.4. A comparison of

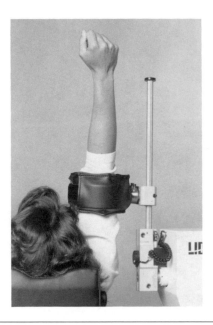

Figure 5.8   Test and exercise position for the shoulder flexor muscles with the resistance pad placed at the distal humerus.

dominant/nondominant bilateral strength in Table 5.3 indicates that nondominant strength of the flexors and extensors is within 5% to 10% of the dominant side musculature. However, remember to consider that selected overuse of the dominant side muscles may influence "normal" bilateral strength relationships.

Shoulder Abduction and Adduction

Shoulder abduction and adduction occur through the coronal, or frontal, plane of the body (Figure 5.9, a and b). Abduction beyond the horizontal plane impinges the greater tubercle of the humerus against the acromion process of the scapula and its underlying soft tissue structures. Outward rotation of the humerus during this phase of abduction enables additional movement by posteriorly displacing the greater tubercle relative to the acromion process. Abduction is accomplished primarily by the combined actions of the deltoid muscle and the rotator cuff (subscapularis, supraspinatus, infraspinatus, and teres minor) musculature. Indeed, the role of the rotator cuff in "depressing" or "pulling inward" the head of the humerus is essential to the success of the deltoid in producing shoulder abduction. Also noteworthy is the importance of scapular movement in permitting this and all other glenohumeral motions. For example, abduction of the glenohumeral joint is

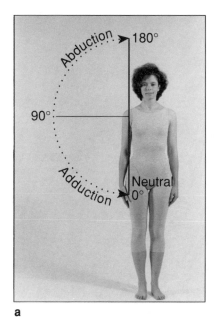

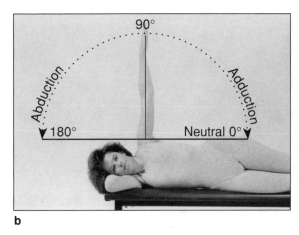

a   b

Figure 5.9   Shoulder abduction and adduction ranges of motion while standing (a) and while laying on side (b).

accompanied by outward rotation of the scapula, especially beyond 40 deg of abduction. Any significant compromise of scapular movement will make isokinetic assessment of the glenohumeral joint through a full range of motion impossible. Adduction of the glenohumeral joint is produced by the sternal portion of the pectoralis major, teres major, and latissimus dorsi muscles. Figure 5.10, a and b illustrates typical subject positioning for assessment of the shoulder abductor and adductor muscles. As with shoulder flexion and extension, better isolation of the shoulder abductors and adductors would probably be accomplished with the resistance pad placed at the distal humerus (Figure 5.11). If you wish to assess or exercise shoulder abduction beyond the horizontal plane, make provisions to permit simultaneous outward rotation of the humerus to preclude the complications associated with shoulder impingement syndrome. Normative isokinetic strength values for the shoulder abductor and adductor muscle groups are presented in Table 5.5.

The shoulder abduction/adduction reciprocal muscle group ratios presented in Table 5.6 indicate the shoulder abductors typically produce 50% to 65% of the torque values generated by the adductor muscles. Comparisons of the shoulder abductor and adductor muscle groups from the values in Table 5.5 indicate a bilateral relationship usually within 5%.

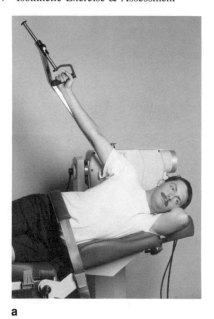
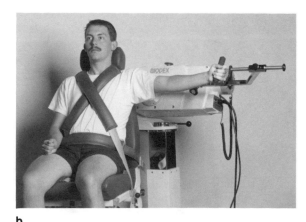

a   b

Figure 5.10   Test and exercise position for the shoulder abductor and adductor muscles while laying on side (a) and seated (b). Exercise beyond 90 deg of shoulder abduction is contradindicated for patients predisposed to shoulder impingement syndrome.

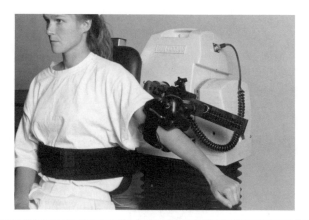

Figure 5.11   Test and exercise position for the shoulder abductor and adductor muscles with the resistance pad placed at the distal humerus.

Shoulder Horizontal Adduction and Abduction

Shoulder horizontal adduction (flexion) and abduction (extension) occur through the transverse plane (Figure 5.12). Horizontal adduction is produced primarily by the sternal and clavicular portions of the pectoralis major and the coracobrachialis muscles. Horizontal abduction is produced by the middle and posterior portions of the deltoid and the infraspinatus and teres minor muscles. Table 5.7 presents the limited normative data for these movements, and Figure 5.13 illustrates a position for testing and exercise through horizontal adduction and abduction. Because a considerable amount of horizontal adduction and abduction occurs against and with the force of gravity, respectively, gravity correction is important to accurately interpret the torque and reciprocal ratios of these muscles. Additional normative data are needed for these muscle groups in a variety of normal and athletic populations.

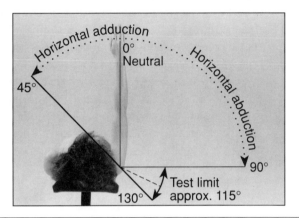

Figure 5.12   Shoulder horizontal adduction and abduction ranges of motion in the supine position.

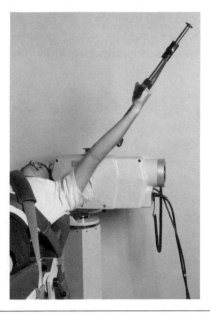

Figure 5.13   Test and exercise position for the shoulder horizontal adductor and abductor muscles.

Modified Shoulder Exercise Positions

The multiple degrees of motion and freedom of movement at the glenohumeral joint permit use of the surrounding muscles from a variety of positions for activities of daily living and athletic participation. Modifications in dynamometer and subject positioning enable exercise of the shoulder musculature from several positions (Soderberg & Blaschak, 1987). For example, in addition to exercising the subject's shoulder internal and external rotators from the adducted (neutral) position, 45 deg abducted, or 90 deg abducted positions (Figure 5.4, a-c), you may also want to rotate the patient to face the dynamometer to perform these exercises with the shoulder horizontally adducted (flexed) to 90 deg (Figure 5.14). These variations enable exercise of the shoulder rotator musculature from a variety of length-tension positions. The nature of injury to a patient will dictate which of these positions is most appropriate. For example, patients experiencing impingement syndrome should avoid exercise from the 90 deg abducted position. Surgical repair for anterior dislocation of the glenohumeral joint also reduces the normal range of shoulder abduction and external rotation. These patients benefit from exercising the shoulder rotator muscles from a position between the plane of the scapula and 90 deg of horizontal adduction. They should also follow a progression of exercise from the neutral (adducted) position to one approaching 90 deg of abduction.

Most isokinetic dynamometers may also be used to isolate specific muscles or muscle groups. For example, the supraspinatus muscle may be isolated by horizontally adducting the shoulder 30 deg and inwardly rotating the humerus until the thumb is turned down. Accomplish this by rotating the patient relative to the dynamometer and modifying the handgrip accessory (Knoeppel, 1985b). Isokinetic exercise may then focus on the supraspinatus during movements of eccentric adduction and concentric abduction (Figure 5.15).

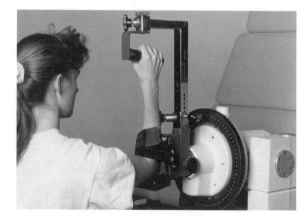

Figure 5.14   Exercise of the shoulder internal and external rotators from 90 deg of horizontal adduction.

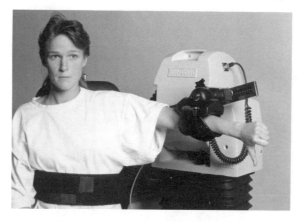

Figure 5.15   Modified exercise position for isolation of the supraspinatus muscle. Note the thumb turned down position combined with 30 deg of horizontal adduction of the shoulder.

THE ELBOW JOINT

The capsule of the elbow joint encloses the articulations of the distal humerus and proximal ulna, the distal humerus and proximal radius, and the proximal aspects of the radius and ulna. The radius and ulna are joined along their respective shafts by the interosseous membrane and end by the formation of the distal radio-ulnar joint. The movements about these articulations include flexion and extension at the humero-ulnar joint, and pronation and supination at the radio-ulnar joints.

Elbow Flexion and Extension

Flexion and extension of the elbow occur through the sagittal plane (Figure 5.16, a and b). Flexion is produced principally by the biceps brachii, brachialis, and brachioradialis muscles. The biceps brachii is the only three-joint muscle in the body, crossing the glenohumeral, humero-ulnar, and proximal radio-ulnar joints; its relative contribution to flexion of the elbow can be altered by changes in position of the shoulder joint. Moreover, by virtue of its distal attachment to the radius, the amount of pronation and supination of the forearm affects the contribution of the biceps brachii in producing flexion of the elbow. The length-tension theory seems to support greater involvement of the biceps brachii as an elbow flexor as the amount of forearm pronation is increased. However, extreme pronation of the forearm places the tendon of the biceps brachii muscle in a disadvantageous mechanical position as it wraps around the radius. As such, the contribution of the biceps brachii to elbow flexion is reduced during extreme pronation of the elbow. You can probably achieve greater isolation of the biceps brachii for isokinetic

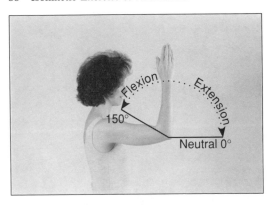
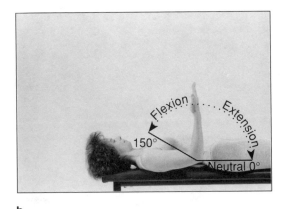

a   b

Figure 5.16   Elbow flexion and extension ranges of motion in the standing (a) and supine (b) positions.

assessment and exercise by placing the forearm in the midposition of pronation and supination.

In contrast to the biceps brachii muscle, the brachialis originates from the
humerus and thus is a one-joint muscle acting exclusively on the humero-
ulnar articulation. Moreover, by virtue of its distal attachment to the ulna,
variations in the amount of forearm pronation and supination have no effect
on the contribution of the brachialis as an elbow flexor. As such, the brachialis
muscle is regarded as the true workhorse in the production of elbow flexion,
regardless of the position of the shoulder or forearm (Basmajian, 1979).
However, because the midposition of forearm pronation and supination places
the biceps brachii and brachioradialis muscles at their optimum positions
for producing elbow flexion, the greatest isolation of the brachialis is probably
achieved by fully supinating the forearm during flexion of the humero-ulnar
joint. To achieve optimal isolation of the three primary elbow flexors, I
recommend variations in the amount of forearm pronation and supination
during exercise of this muscle group.

Extension of the elbow is produced by the triceps brachii muscle. The
long head of the triceps muscle crosses the posterior shoulder joint in addition
to the elbow, so the efficiency of the triceps in producing elbow extension
can be enhanced by increasing the amount of flexion of the shoulder joint.
Figures 5.17 and 5.18 illustrate two positions for exercise and assessment
of the elbow joint.

Table 5.8 presents normal isokinetic strength values for the elbow flexors
and extensors for a variety of populations. Although few studies have reported
bilateral relationships for these muscle groups, little difference is usually
found between the dominant and nondominant sides for either the elbow
flexors or extensors. Reports of the elbow flexor/extensor reciprocal muscle
group relationship are also sparse. A comparison of elbow flexor and extensor

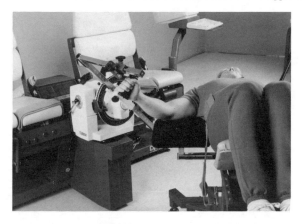

Figure 5.17   Test and exercise position for the elbow flexor and extensor muscles with the shoulder in the neutral position.

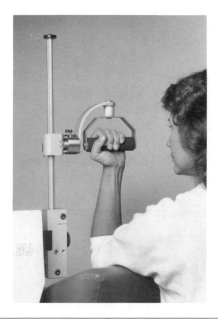

Figure 5.18   Test and exercise position for the elbow flexor and extensor muscles with the shoulder in 90 deg of flexion. This position places the triceps long head in a lengthened position and the biceps brachii in a shortened position.

strength from one study indicates a flexion/extension reciprocal muscle group ratio usually greater than .90 (Table 5.9).

Forearm Pronation and Supination

Pronation and supination of the forearm occur through the transverse plane (Figure 5.19). Forearm pronation and supination with the elbow in complete

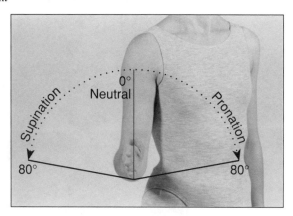

Figure 5.19   Forearm pronation and supination ranges of motion. Isolation of this motion is best accomplished by placing the elbow in 90 deg of flexion to eliminate glenohumeral rotation.

extension are usually accompanied by some degree of shoulder internal and external rotation; true isolation of pronation and supination is best accomplished with the elbow in 90 deg of flexion. The pronator teres and pronator quadratus muscles are the primary movers for forearm pronation. The pronator quadratus is located between the radius and ulna at the distal forearm while the pronator teres crosses the medial aspect of the elbow joint. The respective attachments of these two muscles dictate that the pronator quadratus is not affected by variations in position of the elbow joint, while the pronator teres becomes more involved as a pronator as the elbow moves from flexion to extension. As such, isolation of the pronator quadratus for isokinetic exercise and assessment is best accomplished with the elbow positioned at 90 deg of flexion (Figure 5.20).

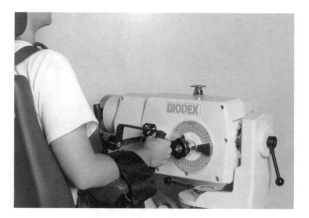

Figure 5.20   Test and exercise position for the forearm pronator and supinator muscles with the elbow in 90 deg of flexion.

Repositioning of the elbow to 120 to 135 deg will enhance the length-tension relationship of the pronator teres and thus increase its involvement in production of elbow pronation (Figure 5.21). Supination of the forearm is accomplished primarily through contraction of the supinator muscle. The biceps brachii muscle is also involved as a supinator, particularly when the elbow is in a flexed position.

Virtually no studies report normal strength values for the pronator and supinator muscles. Additional research is needed to establish normal bilateral and reciprocal muscle group strength relationships for these muscles in a variety of athletic and nonathletic populations.

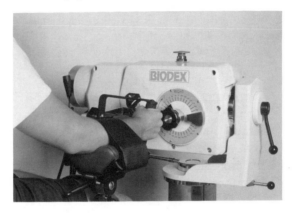

Figure 5.21   Test and exercise position for the forearm pronator and supinator muscles with the elbow in 120-135 deg of flexion.

THE WRIST JOINT

The wrist joint is comprised of the articulation of the distal radius and the scaphoid, lunate, and triquetral bones, and the intercarpal articulation between the proximal and distal rows of carpal bones. The combined movements at these joints permit flexion and extension of the wrist as well as radial deviation (abduction) and ulnar deviation (adduction).

Wrist Flexion and Extension

Flexion and extension of the wrist occur through the sagittal plane (Figure 5.22, a and b) and may be performed with the forearm in the pronated, mid, or supinated position. The primary movers for flexion include the flexor carpi radialis and flexor carpi ulnaris muscles. The major movers for extension include the extensor carpi radialis longus and brevis muscles and the extensor carpi ulnaris muscle. The flexors originate from the medial epicondyle of the humerus, and the extensors originate at or near the lateral epicondyle of the humerus. Pronation of the forearm tends to lengthen the wrist

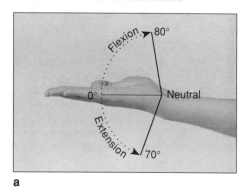
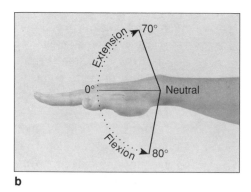

a   b

Figure 5.22 Wrist flexion and extension range of motion with the forearm in the supinated (a) and pronated (b) positions.

extensor muscles and supination tends to lengthen the wrist flexor muscles. The length-tension relationship of the wrist flexor and extensor muscle groups would seem to support the idea that the wrist flexors should produce greater torque from the supinated position than from the pronated position. Conversely, the wrist extensor muscle group should produce greater torque from the pronated position than from the supinated position. However, isokinetic assessment seems not to support the length-tension phenomenon for these muscle groups (VanSwearingen, 1983). Figure 5.23, a and b illustrates recommended positions for assessment of wrist flexion and extension strength.

Table 5.10 presents the limited normative data that may be found for wrist flexor and extensor strength in the scientific literature. The wrist flexor muscle group produces greater peak torque with the forearm in the pronated position than the supinated position. Conversely, the extensor muscle group produces greater peak torque with the forearm in the supinated position. The

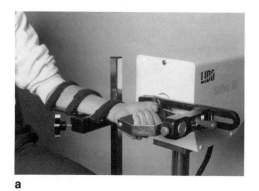
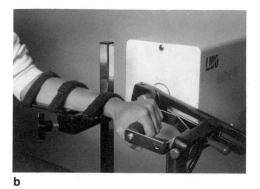

a   b

Figure 5.23 Test and exercise position for the wrist flexor and extensor muscles with the forearm supinated (a) and pronated (b).

dominant side strength is slightly greater than the nondominant side, and the wrist extensor/flexor reciprocal muscle group ratio is on average approximately 55% to 60%.

Wrist Radial and Ulnar Deviation

Radial and ulnar deviation of the wrist occur through the frontal plane (Figure 5.24) and may be performed with the forearm in pronation, supination, or anywhere in between. Radial deviation is performed by the simultaneous contraction of the flexor carpi radialis and extensor carpi radialis longus and brevis muscles. Ulnar deviation results from contraction of the flexor carpi ulnaris and extensor carpi ulnaris muscles. You can best assess radial and ulnar deviation with the wrist in a neutral position, between flexion and extension. See Figure 5.25 for a recommended setup for isokinetic assessment of the wrist radial and ulnar deviator muscle groups.

Table 5.11 presents the limited normative data for wrist radial and ulnar deviation. As with the wrist flexors and extensors, the dominant side strength is greater than the nondominant side. Also, the ulnar deviator muscles tend to produce approximately 80% to 85% of the torque values generated by the radial deviator muscles.

The strength of the forearm pronators and supinators and wrist flexor and extensor muscle groups plays a prominent role in many occupational (e.g., carpentry) and recreational (e.g., tennis) activities. However, limited normative isokinetic strength data are available for these muscle groups. Additional research is needed to establish normal bilateral and reciprocal muscle group strength ratios in a variety of occupational and athletic populations.

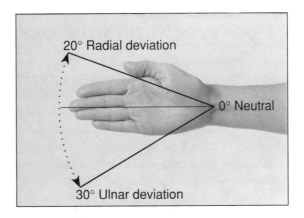

Figure 5.24   Wrist radial and ulnar deviation range of motion.

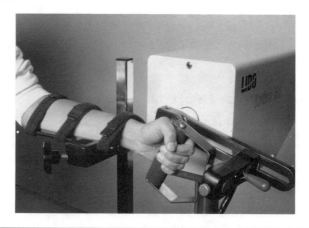

Figure 5.25   Test and exercise position for the wrist radial and ulnar deviator muscles with the forearm in the midposition of pronation and supination.

FUNCTIONAL MOVEMENT PATTERNS

Proprioceptive neuromuscular facilitation (PNF) is a valuable adjunct to rehabilitation of a variety of upper extremity injuries. PNF uses diagonal movement patterns of flexion/abduction/external rotation and extension/adduction/internal rotation to restore normal neuromuscular strength and coordination. Isokinetic dynamometry cannot incorporate all of the features of PNF (e.g., stretch/reflex). However, modifications in dynamometer and subject positioning can sometimes enable replication of some of these functional patterns (Day, Moore, & Patterson, 1988). Figure 5.26, a and b illustrates an upper extremity diagonal movement pattern on an isokinetic dynamometer. As with PNF, these exercises may be valuable adjuncts to isokinetic exercise, which is usually isolated to the traditional cardinal planes of movement.

RELIABILITY OF UPPER EXTREMITY ASSESSMENT

Isokinetic assessment of upper extremity muscle groups is quite reliable. In general, motions that are easily isolated tend to produce higher reliability coefficients than those permitting involvement of accessory muscle groups. For example, reliability of shoulder internal and external rotation tends to be slightly higher than shoulder flexion and extension, probably because of muscles acting on the hand and elbow during contraction of the shoulder flexors and extensors. The reliability of shoulder flexion and extension with resistance pad placement at the distal humerus might produce higher coefficients than when the hand serves as the point of resistance.

Reliability coefficients also tend to be higher during assessment of concentric peak torque than during eccentric peak torque. Novice subjects seem to

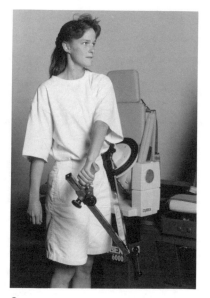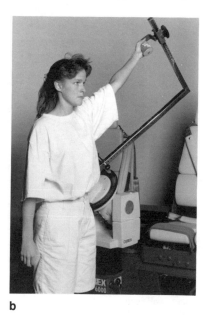

a   **b**

Figure 5.26   Modified position designed to exercise the upper extremity through a diagonal pattern from low (a) to high (b).

have more motor control difficulty during eccentric contractions than during concentric contractions, particularly at higher test velocities. This point seems to support the need for a longer familiarization period during assessment of eccentric peak torque.

Table 5.12 summarizes several published reports of reliability during isokinetic assessment of several upper extremity muscle groups. In making comparisons with the coefficients in this table, carefully consider the subject population, the test position (particularly with respect to the glenohumeral joint), and the isokinetic dynamometer used for assessment of peak torque. In addition, these studies utilized either a Pearson product-moment correlation or an intraclass correlation coefficient to estimate reliability of measurement. The Pearson product-moment correlation, a bivariate statistic, is best utilized when X and Y scores represent different variables rather than repeated administrations of the same test (Safrit & Wood, 1989). On the other hand, the intraclass correlation coefficient, a univariate statistic, is the preferred technique for estimating reliability of repeated measures (Safrit & Wood, 1989). Each of the reliability tables in this text indicate which of these two statistical techniques was used to estimate reliability of measurement.

Table 5.1

Table 5.1
Normative Values of Shoulder Internal and External Rotation Peak Torque (in ft-lb)

Study and population	Sex	Age	Dominant internal rotation	Non-dominant internal rotation	Dominant external rotation	Non-dominant external rotation
30 deg/s						
McMaster et al. (1991)						
Nondisabled (neutral adduction)	M	22	39.3	36.8	29.1	28.1
National water polo team (neutral adduction)	M	26	65.9	57.8	38.2	34.8
McMaster et al. (1992)						
Nondisabled (neutral adduction)	M	22	39.3	36.8	29.1	28.1
	F	23	27.2	26.7	20.3	20.1
Competitive swimmers (neutral adduction)	M	20	66.8	55.9	33.7	31.8
	F	18.5	41.5	37.6	26.0	23.4
48 deg/s						
Otis et al. (1990)						
Nondisabled (90 deg abduction) (GC)	M	26	31.3	28.0	24.6	24.0
60 deg/s						
Ivey et al. (1985)						
Mixed exercisers and nonexercisers (90 deg abduction)	M	27	36.4		23.8	
	F	27	19.6		13.9	
Walmsley & Szybbo (1987)						
Nondisabled (90 deg abduction)	F	19-25	18.3		14.1	
Pawlowski & Perrin (1989)						
College pitchers (90 deg abduction)	M	20	41.1		27.2	
Hageman et al. (1989)						
Nondisabled (45 deg abduction)	M	21-33	35.8		22.6	
		(E)	40.5		25.1	
	F	21-33	17.5		12.0	
		(E)	21.5		13.4	
Connelly Maddux et al. (1989)						
Nondisabled (90 deg abduction)	M	34	42.0	39.0	26.0	24.0
	F	26	17.0	17.0	11.0	12.0

Table 5.1 *(continued)*

Study and population	Sex	Age	Dominant internal rotation	Non-dominant internal rotation	Dominant external rotation	Non-dominant external rotation
Hellwig & Perrin (1991)						
Nondisabled (90 deg abduction	M	21		29.5		19.5
90 deg/s						
Alderink & Kuck (1986)						
High school and college pitchers (90 deg abduction)	M	18	39.1	38.4	26.3	26.8
Hinton (1988)						
High school pitchers (90 deg abduction)	M	16	29.1	25.7	19.8	19.3
120 deg/s						
Alderink & Kuck (1986)						
High school and college pitchers (90 deg abduction)	M	18	37.3	36.2	25.1	26.0
Walmsley & Szybbo (1987)						
Nondisabled (90 deg abduction)	F	19-25	17.3		13.1	
180 deg/s						
Ivey et al. (1985)						
Mixed exercisers and	M	27	32.7		21.1	
nonexercisers (90 deg abduction)	F	27	17.1		11.2	
Walmsley & Szybbo (1987)						
Nondisabled (90 deg abduction)	F	19-25	17.0		12.4	
Brown et al. (1988)						
Major league baseball pitchers (neutral adduction)	M	27	42.5	38.9	28.2	28.1
Hageman et al. (1989)						
Nondisabled (45 deg abduction)	M	21-33	31.2		19.7	
		(E)	39.9		24.8	
	F	21-33	16.4		11.4	
		(E)	21.1		14.7	

(continued)

Table 5.1 *(continued)*

Study and population	Sex	Age	Dominant internal rotation	Non-dominant internal rotation	Dominant external rotation	Non-dominant external rotation
Connelly Maddux et al. (1989)						
Nondisabled (90 deg abduction)	M	34	32.0	30.0	19.0	18.0
	F	26	14.0	13.0	9.0	8.0
McMaster et al. (1991)						
Nondisabled (neutral adduction)	M	22	41.8	37.6	27.4	25.4
National water polo team (neutral adduction)	M	26	65.9	55.8	34.5	30.5
McMaster et al. (1992)						
Nondisabled (neutral adduction)	M	22	41.8	37.6	27.4	25.4
	F	23	27.9	27.6	16.5	18.2
Competitive swimmers	M	20	66.3	52.1	28.4	27.4
(neutral adduction)	F	18.5	33.8	30.7	18.5	18.7
210 deg/s						
Alderink & Kuck (1986)						
High school and college	M	18	33.2	33.2	23.5	25.2
240 deg/s						
Brown et al. (1988)						
Major league baseball pitchers (neutral adduction)	M	27	40.5	36.3	25.0	24.1
Hinton (1988)						
High school pitchers (90 deg abduction)	M	16	20.4	18.5	14.5	14.5
Pawlowski & Perrin (1989)						
College pitchers (90 deg abduction)	M	20	29.5		20.4	
300 deg/s						
Alderink & Kuck (1986)						
High school and college pitchers (90 deg abduction)	M	18	31.7	31.3	22.1	23.6
Brown et al. (1988)						
Major league baseball pitchers (neutral adduction)	M	27	38.7	33.1	22.8	21.5

Note. GC—gravity correction procedure used; E—eccentric (position of glenohumeral joint during testing).

Table 5.2
Normative Values of Shoulder External/Internal Rotation Reciprocal Muscle Group Ratios (Percent)

Study and population	Sex	Age	Dominant external rotation/internal rotation	Nondominant external rotation/internal rotation
30 deg/s				
McMaster et al. (1991)				
Nondisabled (neutral adduction)	M	22	.74	.78
National water polo team (neutral adduction)	M	26	.61	.61
60 deg/s				
Connelly Maddux et al. (1989)				
Nondisabled (90 deg abduction)	M	34	.63	.62
	F	26	.70	.71
90 deg/s				
Alderink & Kuck (1986)				
High school and college pitchers (90 deg abduction)	M	18	.66	.70
Hinton (1988)				
High school pitchers (90 deg abduction)	M	16	.69	.76
120 deg/s				
Alderink & Kuck (1986)				
High school and college pitchers (90 deg abduction)	M	18	.68	.72
180 deg/s				
Cook et al. (1987)				
College baseball pitchers (90 deg abduction)	M	18-25	.70	.81
Age-matched nonpitchers (90 deg abduction)	M	18-25	.83	.78
Brown et al. (1988)				
Major league baseball pitchers (neutral adduction)	M	27	.67	.71

(continued)

Table 5.2 *(continued)*

Study and population	Sex	Age	Dominant external rotation/internal rotation	Nondominant external rotation/internal rotation
Connelly Maddux et al. (1989)				
Nondisabled (90 deg abduction)	M	34	.61	.63
	F	26	.64	.68
McMaster et al. (1991)				
Nondisabled (neutral adduction)	M	22	.65	.66
National water polo team (neutral adduction)	M	26	.55	.56
210 deg/s				
Alderink & Kuck (1986)				
High school and college pitchers (90 deg abduction)	M	18	.71	.76
240 deg/s				
Brown et al. (1988)				
Major league baseball pitchers (neutral adduction)	M	27	.61	.66
Hinton (1988)				
High school pitchers (90 deg abduction)	M	16	.71	.80
300 deg/s				
Alderink & Kuck (1986)				
High school and college pitchers (90 deg abduction)	M	18	.70	.76
Cook et al. (1987)				
College baseball pitchers (90 deg abduction)	M	18-25	.70	.81
Age-matched nonpitchers (90 deg abduction)	M	18-25	.87	.79
Brown et al. (1988)				
Major league baseball pitchers (neutral adduction)	M	27	.65	.65

Table 5.3

Table 5.3
Normative Values of Shoulder Flexion and Extension Peak Torque (in ft-lb)

Study and population	Sex	Age	Dominant flexion	Nondominant flexion	Dominant extension	Nondominant extension
15 deg/s						
Tesch (1983)						
Kayakers	M	22			59.0	
Bodybuilders	M	24			73.8	
Water-skiers	M	22			59.0	
30 deg/s						
Weltman et al. (1988)						
Prepubertal boys (values expressed as mean work output)	M	6-11	21.6	20.7	32.1	32.5
60 deg/s						
Tesch (1983)						
Kayakers	M	22			53.1	
Bodybuilders	M	24			62.7	
Water-skiers	M	22			56.0	
Ivey et al. (1985)						
Mixed exercisers and	M	27	45.8		59.1	
nonexercisers	F	27	26.2		31.6	
Berg et al. (1985)						
College basketball players	F	20	34.5	33.4	44.5	41.4
Pawlowski & Perrin (1989)						
College pitchers	M	20	48.1		66.6	
Nicholas et al. (1989)						
Nondisabled	M	20-30	57.0		39.0	
	F	20-30	28.0		18.0	
90 deg/s						
Alderink & Kuck (1986)						
High school and college pitchers	M	18	43.2	42.7	82.7	76.7
Weltman et al. (1988)						
Prepubertal boys (values expressed as mean work output)	M	6-11	18.0	17.1	27.3	27.6

(continued)

Table 5.3 *(continued)*

Study and population	Sex	Age	Dominant flexion	Nondominant flexion	Dominant extension	Nondominant extension
120 deg/s						
Berg et al. (1985)						
College basketball players	F	20	31.9	30.6	40.2	38.6
Alderink & Kuck (1986)						
High school and college pitchers	M	18	40.7	39.7	77.2	72.3
180 deg/s						
Tesch (1983)						
Kayakers	M	22			47.9	
Bodybuilders	M	24			47.2	
Water-skiers	M	22			49.4	
Ivey et al. (1985)						
Mixed exercisers and	M	27	37.5		47.6	
nonexercisers	F	27	28.8		24.8	
Berg et al. (1985)						
College basketball players	F	20	28.7	28.0	34.2	34.1
Nicholas et al. (1989)						
Nondisabled	M	20-30	49.0		30.0	
	F	20-30	19.0		11.0	
210 deg/s						
Alderink & Kuck (1986)						
High school and college pitchers	M	18	34.7	32.2	67.3	62.4
240 deg/s						
Berg et al. (1985)						
College basketball players	F	20	23.7	23.9	29.1	29.4
Pawlowski & Perrin (1989)						
College pitchers	M	20	34.6		46.6	
300 deg/s						
Berg et al. (1985)						
College basketball players	F	20	18.3	18.3	22.4	22.8
Alderink & Kuck (1986)						
High school and college pitchers	M	18	28.2	26.5	57.9	54.3

Table 5.4
Normative Values of Shoulder Flexion/Extension Reciprocal Muscle Group Ratios (Percent)

Study and population	Sex	Age	Dominant flexion/extension	Nondominant flexion/extension
60 deg/s				
Berg et al. (1985)				
College basketball players	F	18-22	.77	.81
90 deg/s				
Alderink & Kuck (1986)				
High school and college pitchers	M	18	.52	.55
120 deg/s				
Berg et al. (1985)				
College basketball players	F	18-22	.80	.79
Alderink & Kuck (1986)				
High school and college pitchers	M	18	.52	.55
180 deg/s				
Berg et al. (1985)				
College basketball players	F	18-22	.84	.82
Cook et al. (1987)				
College baseball pitchers	M	18-25	.74	.81
Age-matched nonpitchers	M	18-25	.91	.86
210 deg/s				
Alderink & Kuck (1986)				
High school and college pitchers	M	18	.51	.51
240 deg/s				
Berg et al. (1985)				
College basketball players	F	18-22	.81	.81
300 deg/s				
Berg et al. (1985)				
College basketball players	F	18-22	.82	.80
Alderink & Kuck (1986)				
High school and college pitchers	M	18	.48	.48
Cook et al. (1987)				
College baseball pitchers	M	18-25	.70	.71
Age-matched nonpitchers	M	18-25	.99	.76

Table 5.5

Table 5.5
Normative Values of Shoulder Abduction and Adduction Peak Torque (in ft-lb)

Study and population	Sex	Age	Dominant abduction	Nondominant abduction	Dominant adduction	Nondominant adduction
			30 deg/s			
Smith et al. (1981) Professional and elite amateur ice hockey players	M	24	55.5		78.5	
Smith et al. (1982) Canadian Olympic hockey team	M	22	51.6		76.0	
McMaster et al. (1991)						
Nondisabled	M	22	35.3	38.2	54.0	52.7
National water polo team	M	26	51.8	49.4	99.1	92.7
McMaster et al. (1992)						
Nondisabled	M	22	35.3	38.2	54.0	52.7
	F	23	24.2	25.4	39.9	40.3
Competitive swimmers	M	20	48.1	48.6	99.1	102.2
	F	18.5	27.5	29.5	57.2	58.0
			48 deg/s			
Otis et al. (1990) Nondisabled	M	26	36.7	34.3		
			60 deg/s			
Ivey et al. (1985) Mixed exercisers and	M	27	41.6		65.9	
nonexercisers	F	27	21.6		37.2	
Connelly Maddux et al. (1989) Nondisabled (test position	M	34	39.0	37.0	63.0	60.0
modified for isolation of supraspinatus muscle)	F	27	19.0	19.0	32.0	30.0
			90 deg/s			
Alderink & Kuck (1986) High school and college pitchers	M	18	47.8	46.6	87.5	80.4

Table 5.5 *(continued)*

Study and population	Sex	Age	Dominant abduction	Nondominant abduction	Dominant adduction	Nondominant adduction
			120 deg/s			
Alderink & Kuck (1986)						
High school and college pitchers	M	18	45.0	44.9	82.7	78.6
			180 deg/s			
Smith et al. (1981)						
Professional and elite amateur ice hockey players	M	24	43.2		58.8	
Smith et al. (1982)						
Canadian Olympic hockey team	M	22	41.8		56.9	
Ivey et al. (1985)						
Mixed exercisers and	M	27	31.2		55.5	
nonexercisers	F	27	15.5		30.7	
Connelly Maddux et al. (1989)						
Nondisabled (test position	M	34	24.0	25.0	53.0	47.0
modified for isolation of	F	27	15.0	15.0	23.0	21.0
supraspinatus muscle)						
McMaster et al. (1991)						
Nondisabled	M	22	32.6	35.2	47.6	55.9
National water polo team	M	26	45.7	44.4	91.0	87.0
McMaster et al. (1992)						
Nondisabled	M	22	32.6	35.2	47.6	55.9
	F	23	22.5	22.0	39.0	38.0
Competitive swimmers	M	20	41.8	43.5	92.2	99.3
	F	18.5	18.2	22.2	37.1	46.4
			210 deg/s			
Alderink & Kuck (1986)						
High school and college pitchers	M	18	38.0	37.8	74.4	72.4
			300 deg/s			
Alderink & Kuck (1986)						
High school and college pitchers	M	18	31.4	31.4	61.9	62.7

Table 5.6
Normative Values of Shoulder Abduction/Adduction Reciprocal Muscle Group Ratios (Percent)

Study and population	Sex	Age	Dominant abduction/ adduction	Nondominant abduction/ adduction
30 deg/s				
Smith et al. (1981)				
Professional and elite amateur ice hockey players	M	24	.73	
60 deg/s				
Connelly Maddux et al. (1989)				
Nondisabled (test position modified	M	34	.66	.65
for isolation of supraspinatus muscle)	F	27	.61	.66
90 deg/s				
Alderink & Kuck (1986)				
High school and college pitchers	M	18	.54	.57
120 deg/s				
Alderink & Kuck (1986)				
High school and college pitchers	M	18	.54	.57
180 deg/s				
Smith et al. (1981)				
Professional and elite amateur ice hockey players	M	24	.76	
Connelly Maddux et al. (1989)				
Nondisabled (test position modified	M	34	.49	.56
for isolation of supraspinatus muscle)	F	27	.74	.82
210 deg/s				
Alderink & Kuck (1986)				
High school and college pitchers	M	18	.50	.52
300 deg/s				
Alderink & Kuck (1986)				
High school and college pitchers	M	18	.51	.50

Table 5.7
Normative Values of Shoulder Horizontal Abduction and Adduction Peak Torque (in ft-lb)

Study and population	Sex	Age	Dominant abduction	Dominant adduction
30 deg/s				
Weir et al. (1992)				
High school wrestlers	M	<15	42.4	43.3
		15-16	46.9	46.7
		16-17	48.7	56.2
		>17	52.5	57.2
180 deg/s				
Weir et al. (1992)				
High school wrestlers	M	<15	30.6	29.4
		15-16	34.6	31.5
		16-17	37.8	37.0
		>17	38.7	42.0
300 deg/s				
Weir et al. (1992)				
High school wrestlers	M	<15	21.1	20.2
		15-16	24.8	22.6
		16-17	26.2	24.0
		>17	27.1	27.1

Table 5.8

Table 5.8
Normative Values of Elbow Flexion and Extension Peak Torque (in ft-lb)

Study and population	Sex	Age	Dominant flexion	Nondominant flexion	Dominant extension	Nondominant extension
30 deg/s						
Gilliam et al. (1979)						
Active children (Dom =	M	7-13	9.5		12.9	
average of right and left	F	7-13	8.6		12.3	
sides adjusted [ANCOVA]						
for age)						
Griffin (1987)						
Athletic and sedentary	F	27	25.1			
		(E)	28.0			
Weltman et al. (1988)						
Prepubertal boys (values	M	6-11	14.1	14.6	15.6	14.6
expressed as mean work						
output)						
Hortobagyi & Katch (1990)						
Weight-trained subjects	M	23	51.4		60.1	
		(E)	69.5		73.9	
Non-weight-trained subjects	M	23	37.3		41.5	
		(E)	53.7		54.9	
60 deg/s						
Berg et al. (1985)						
College basketball players	F	20	26.5	26.3	29.4	30.5
Pawlowski & Perrin (1989)						
College pitchers	M	20	42.6		41.5	
90 deg/s						
Weltman et al. (1988)						
Prepubertal boys (values	M	6-11	12.6	13.2	14.0	11.8
expressed as mean work						
output)						
Hortobagyi & Katch (1990)						
Weight-trained subjects	M	23	48.7		52.7	
		(E)	71.7		77.7	
Non-weight-trained subjects	M	23	36.4		39.7	
		(E)	55.0		55.6	

Table 5.8 *(continued)*

Study and population	Sex	Age	Dominant flexion	Nondominant flexion	Dominant extension	Nondominant extension
			120 deg/s			
Gilliam et al. (1979)						
Active children (average of	M	7-13	8.6		11.3	
right and left sides adjusted	F	7-13	7.4		10.4	
[ANCOVA] for age)						
Berg et al. (1985)						
College basketball players	F	20	23.4	22.8	22.8	24.2
Griffin (1987)						
Athletic and sedentary	F	27	22.2			
		(E)	28.8			
Hortobagyi & Katch (1990)						
Weight-trained subjects	M	23	47.0		51.3	
		(E)	75.5		78.7	
Non-weight-trained subjects	M	23	35.7		37.8	
		(E)	54.8		57.1	
			180 deg/s			
Berg et al. (1985)						
College basketball players	F	20	20.5	19.9	20.4	21.6
			210 deg/s			
Griffin (1987)						
Athletic and sedentary	F	27	19.9			
		(E)	26.3			
			240 deg/s			
Berg et al. (1985)						
College basketball players	F	20	19.7	17.2	18.9	19.2
Pawlowski & Perrin (1989)						
College pitchers	M	20	27.9		29.1	
			300 deg/s			
Berg et al. (1985)						
College basketball players	F	20	16.0	14.7	15.8	15.5

Note. Dom—dominant; ANCOVA—analysis of covariance; E—eccentric.

Table 5.9
Normative Values of Elbow Flexion/Extension Reciprocal Muscle Group Ratios (Percent)

Study and population	Sex	Age	Dominant flexion/extension	Nondominant flexion/extension
Berg et al. (1985)				
College basketball players				
60 deg/s	F	20	.90	.86
120 deg/s	F	20	1.03	.94
180 deg/s	F	20	1.04	.92
240 deg/s	F	20	1.04	.90
300 deg/s	F	20	1.01	.95

Table 5.10
Normative Values of Wrist Flexion and Extension Peak Torque (in ft-lb)

Study and population	Sex	Age	Dominant flexion	Nondominant flexion	Dominant extension	Nondominant extension
			60 deg/s			
VanSwearingen (1983)						
Nondisabled	F and M	22	10.2*	9.4*	5.1[+]	4.6[+]
			7.9[+]	7.6[+]	3.5*	3.3*
Nicholas et al. (1989)						
Nondisabled	M	20-30	4.3		5.7	
	F	20-30	5.7		5.8	
			120 deg/s			
Nicholas et al. (1989)						
Nondisabled	M	20-30	2.6		4.6	
	F	20-30	3.5		2.6	

Note. *—pronated forearm; [+]—supinated forearm.

Table 5.11
Normative Values of Wrist Radial and Ulnar Deviation Peak Torque (in ft-lb)

Study and population	Sex	Age	Dominant radial deviation	Nondominant radial deviation	Dominant ulnar deviation	Nondominant ulnar deviation
60 deg/s						
VanSwearingen (1983) Nondisabled	F and M	22	7.5	6.5	5.6	5.5

Table 5.12
Test-Retest Reliability Coefficients for Upper Extremity Isokinetic Assessment of Peak Torque

Study and population	Velocity (deg/s)	Joint position	Dominant side correlation coefficient	Nondominant side correlation coefficient
Shoulder internal rotation				
Perrin (1986)				
Nondisabled; men; Cybex; (r)	60 (C)	90 deg abduction	.92	.86
	180 (C)	90 deg abduction	.84	.74
Hageman et al. (1989)				
Nondisabled; men and women;	60 (C)	45 deg flexion	.93	
Kin-Com; (r)	60 (E)	45 deg flexion	.90	
	180 (C)	45 deg flexion	.91	
	180 (E)	45 deg flexion	.88	
	60 (C)	45 deg abduction	.92	
	60 (E)	45 deg abduction	.90	
	180 (C)	45 deg abduction	.90	
	180 (E)	45 deg abduction	.88	
Greenfield et al. (1990)				
Nondisabled; men and women; Merac; (r)	60 (C)	45 deg abduction, frontal plane	.92	
	60 (C)	45 deg abduction, scapular plane	.92	
Hellwig & Perrin (1991)				
Nondisabled; men; Kin-Com; (ICC)	60 (C)	90 deg abduction, frontal plane		.90
	60 (E)	90 deg abduction, frontal plane		.94
	60 (C)	90 deg abduction, scapular plane		.89
	60 (E)	90 deg abduction, scapular plane		.80
Shoulder external rotation				
Perrin (1986)				
Nondisabled; men; Cybex; (r)	60 (C)	90 deg abduction	.93	.91
	180 (C)	90 deg abduction	.88	.91

Table 5.12 *(continued)*

Study and population	Velocity (deg/s)	Joint position	Dominant side correlation coefficient	Nondominant side correlation coefficient
Shoulder external rotation				
Hageman et al. (1989)				
Nondisabled; men and women;	60 (C)	45 deg flexion	.90	
Kin-Com; (r)	60 (E)	45 deg flexion	.87	
	180 (C)	45 deg flexion	.89	
	180 (E)	45 deg flexion	.85	
	60 (C)	45 deg abduction	.87	
	60 (E)	45 deg abduction	.85	
	180 (C)	45 deg abduction	.85	
	180 (E)	45 deg abduction	.83	
Greenfield et al. (1990)				
Nondisabled; men and women;	60 (C)	45 deg abduction, frontal plane	.81	
Merac; (r)	60 (C)	45 deg abduction, scapular plane	.94	
Hellwig & Perrin (1991)				
Nondisabled; men; Kin-Com;	60 (C)	90 deg abduction, frontal plane		.93
(ICC)	60 (E)	90 deg abduction, frontal plane		.94
	60 (C)	90 deg abduction, scapular plane		.76
	60 (E)	90 deg abduction, scapular plane		.93
Shoulder flexion				
Perrin (1986)				
Nondisabled; men; Cybex; (r)	60 (C)		.91	.84
	180 (C)		.77	.75
Shoulder extension				
Perrin (1986)				
Nondisabled; men; Cybex; (r)	60 (C)		.92	.95
	180 (C)		.87	.85

(continued)

Table 5.12 *(continued)*

Study and population	Velocity (deg/s)	Joint position	Dominant side correlation coefficient	Nondominant side correlation coefficient
		Elbow flexion		
Griffin (1987)				
Nondisabled; women;	30 (C)	neutral		.83
Kin-Com; (ICC)	30 (E)	neutral		.80
	120 (C)	neutral		.82
	120 (E)	neutral		.72
		Wrist flexion		
VanSwearingen (1983)				
Nondisabled; women and men;	60 (C)	pronated	.99	.98
Cybex; (r)	60 (C)	supinated	.96	.96
		Wrist extension		
VanSwearingen (1983)				
Nondisabled; women and men;	60 (C)	supinated	.95	.89
Cybex; (r)	60 (C)	pronated	.82	.64
		Wrist radial deviation		
VanSwearingen (1983)				
Nondisabled; women and men; Cybex; (r)	60 (C)		.91	.89
		Wrist ulnar deviation		
VanSwearingen (1983)				
Nondisabled; women and men; Cybex; (r)	60 (C)		.92	.86

Note. Joint position denotes position of the glenohumeral joint or forearm during assessment. r—Pearson product-moment correlation coefficient; C—concentric; E—eccentric; ICC—intraclass correlation coefficient.

Chapter 6

Isokinetic Assessment and Exercise of the Lower Extremity

Isokinetic exercise and assessment of the lower extremity, the knee in particular, are of the utmost interest to both clinicians and researchers. In this chapter I describe the muscles acting on the hip, knee, and ankle and discuss patellofemoral and tibiofemoral joint forces, which you will find useful for developing safe isokinetic protocols. I also emphasize the importance of functional and closed-kinetic-chain exercise in the rehabilitation process. The tables at the end of the chapter present the rather expansive normative data for the muscle groups of the lower extremity, with the final table showing the reliability of measuring each of these muscles.

THE HIP JOINT

The hip joint consists of the articulation of the head of the femur and the acetabulum of the innominate bone. This ball-and-socket joint can move through each of the cardinal planes, although the depth and strong supporting capsule of the articulation tend to limit motion compared to the glenohumeral joint of the shoulder. The rather expansive cross-sectional area of the muscles that cross the hip produce the highest levels of isokinetic peak torque found in either the upper or lower extremities.

Hip Flexion and Extension

Flexion and extension of the hip occur through the sagittal plane (see Figure 6.1, a and b). The muscles most involved in producing flexion include the iliopsoas, rectus femoris, and pectineus. Extension is produced by the gluteus maximus and by the biceps femoris, semitendinosus, and semimembranosus

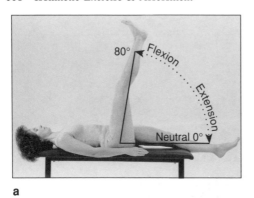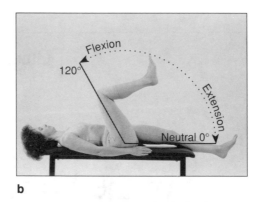

a   **b**

Figure 6.1   Hip flexion and extension ranges of motion from the supine position. Flexion of the hip is limited to approximately 80 deg with the knee in the extended position (a) due to tautness of the hamstring muscle group while range of motion increases to approximately 120° with knee bent (b).

of the hamstring group. The gluteus maximus becomes prominent as an extensor of the hip during heavy or moderate efforts (Rasch, 1989).

Figure 6.2, a and b illustrates a position for exercise and assessment of the hip flexor and extensor muscles. The rectus femoris and hamstring muscles are biarticulate, crossing both hip and knee joints, so you can get a greater magnitude of force by placing these muscles on stretch prior to

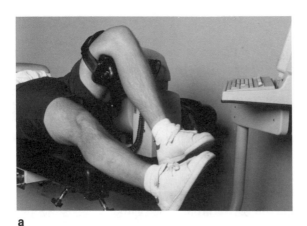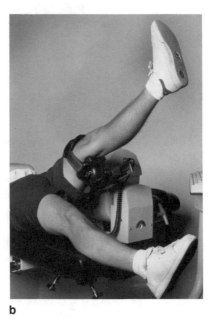

a   **b**

Figure 6.2   Test and exercise position for the hip flexor and extensor muscles while supine with knee bent (a) and straight (b).

contraction. For example, involvement of the rectus femoris as a hip flexor can be enhanced by flexing the knee joint. Conversely, the hamstrings will become more prominently involved in producing hip extension by extending the knee. Optimal isolation of the gluteus maximus occurs by maintaining knee flexion during hip extension. To insure optimal overload of the thigh muscles, exercise of the hip (and knee) should occur from a variety of lengthened and shortened length-tension positions (Knoeppel, 1985a).

Table 6.1 presents normative peak torque values for the hip flexors and extensors. As expected, the substantial cross-sectional area of the gluteus maximus and hamstring muscles produces greater torque values during hip extension than do the hip flexor muscles during hip flexion. Limb dominance tends to have a less pronounced effect on lower extremity than upper extremity muscle groups—bilateral comparisons in the lower extremity are usually within 5% to 10%. The hip flexion/extension reciprocal muscle group ratios listed in Table 6.2 indicate that the flexor musculature produces 60% to 75% of the torque values generated by the extensor muscle group.

Hip Abduction and Adduction

Abduction and adduction of the hip joint occur through the coronal plane of the body (Figure 6.3). Abduction is produced primarily by the gluteus medius, gluteus minimus, and tensor fascia latae muscles. Involvement of the tensor fascia latae muscle may be enhanced by placing the hip in 30 to 45 deg of flexion during abduction. Few activities of daily living or athletic participation require complete abduction of the hip joint; the most important responsibility of this muscle group is likely the role of the gluteus medius in maintaining a level pelvis during the weight-bearing phase of walking (Rasch & Burke, 1978). The major movers for hip adduction

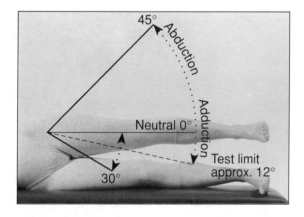

Figure 6.3 Hip abduction and adduction range of motion while laying on side.

are the pectineus, gracilis, and adductor longus, brevis, and magnus muscle group. Interestingly, the fibers of the gluteus maximus located superior to an axis of rotation through the femoral neck (45%-50% of the muscle) assist in abduction of the hip. Conversely, the remaining 50% to 60% of the fibers running obliquely inferior to this axis adduct the hip. Figure 6.4 illustrates the correct position for assessment of hip abductor and adductor muscle group strength. Figure 6.5 illustrates greater isolation of the tensor fascia latae by maintaining flexion of the hip during abduction.

Table 6.3 presents normative values for hip abduction and adduction in both athletic and nondisabled individuals. In contrast to the hip abductors, adduction of this joint is an important component of many athletic activities. As such, the adductor muscle group tends to be substantially stronger than the abductor muscles, although this large discrepancy may be due in part to the absence of a gravity correction procedure in most studies. If hip abduction and adduction are assessed with the subject laying on his or her side, the significant mass of the lower extremity necessitates use of a gravity correction procedure. In this test position, abduction is opposed by gravity and adduction is assisted by gravity (Figure 6.4). The impact of gravity correction would thus be to add to the torque produced by the abductor muscle group and to subtract from that produced by the adductor muscles. Table 6.4 presents the hip abduction/adduction reciprocal muscle group ratios for elite soccer players and nondisabled subjects. The rather large discrepancy in these studies suggests that further research is needed to establish normal reciprocal muscle group ratios (with gravity correction) in a variety of athletic and sedentary populations.

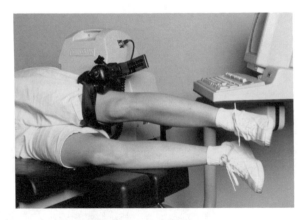

Figure 6.4   Test and exercise position for the hip abductor and adductor muscles while laying on side.

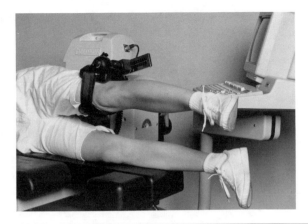

Figure 6.5   Test and exercise position for isolation of the tensor fascia latae muscle while laying on side. Note that the hip is flexed approximately 30 deg during abduction.

Hip Internal and External Rotation

Inward and outward rotation of the hip joint occurs through the transverse plane (Figure 6.6). Inward rotation is produced primarily by the gluteus minimus with assistance from the adductor muscle group. The prime movers for outward rotation are the gluteus maximus, piriformis, obturator internus and externus, gemellus superior and inferior, and the quadratus femoris muscles. There is very little normative isokinetic data for the hip internal and external rotator muscle groups. The values found for college baseball pitchers in Table 6.5 indicate that the internal rotators produce slightly greater torque than the external rotator muscle group. As with hip abduction and adduction, further research is needed to establish normal values of isokinetic internal and external rotation for a variety of populations. Figure 6.7 illustrates a test position for assessment of hip internal and external rotation.

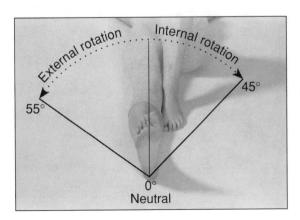

Figure 6.6   Hip internal and external rotation range of motion from the supine position.

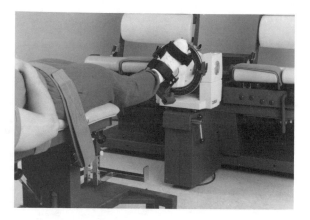

Figure 6.7   Test and exercise position for the hip internal and external rotator muscles with the knee extended while supine.

THE KNEE JOINT

The knee joint is a modified hinge joint formed by the articulation of the distal femur and the proximal tibia. The knee is capable of flexion and extension through the sagittal plane (Figure 6.8, a and b). It is a modified hinge joint in the sense that extension is accompanied by outward rotation of the tibia, and flexion occurs together with inward rotation of the tibia. The anatomical configuration of the knee joint renders it highly vulnerable to injury. A plethora of information in the orthopedic and isokinetic literature addresses the biomechanics and kinesiology of the knee in both healthy and injured populations.

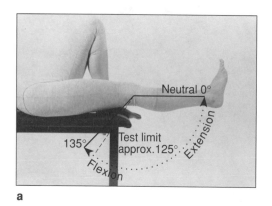
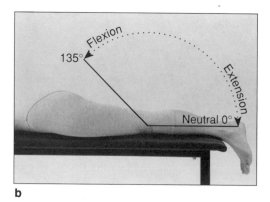

Figure 6.8   Knee extension and flexion range of motion from the supine (a) and prone (b) positions.

Knee Extension and Flexion

No fewer than 12 muscles cross the knee joint, contributing to both its stability and function. Knee extension is accomplished primarily by contraction of the quadriceps femoris muscles, which consist of the rectus femoris and vasti medialis, intermedius, and lateralis muscles (see illustration on p. 72). The rectus femoris is a biarticulate (two-joint) muscle that crosses both the hip and knee. Its prominence in producing knee extension can be enhanced by moving the hip to an extended position, although complete supination tends to place the rectus femoris in an inefficiently lengthened position (Worrell, Perrin, & Denegar, 1989). Knee flexion is produced by the hamstring muscle group, which consists of the biceps femoris, semitendinosus, and semimembranosus muscles. With the exception of the short head of the biceps, each of these muscles crosses the hip joint, so the hamstring muscle group produces less torque during knee flexion when the hip is in an extended position (Figure 6.8, a and b) than from a position of hip flexion (Figure 6.9) (Worrell et al., 1989). The gastrocnemius muscle assists the hamstring muscle group in producing flexion of the knee. The plantaris muscle passes the posterior aspect of the knee as well, but its small cross-sectional area makes it an insignificant contributor to production of knee flexion.

Figure 6.9 illustrates a common position for assessment of the knee extensor and flexor muscles. Although most normative data for these muscle

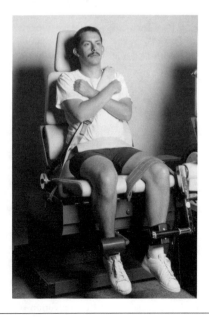

Figure 6.9 Test and exercise position for the knee extensor and flexor muscles while seated. Note arms folded across chest to isolate muscles acting on the knee.

groups have been obtained from the seated position, the alternative positions in Figures 6.10 and 6.11 are also recommended for isokinetic exercise and assessment of the knee extensor and flexor muscles. The hamstring muscles can produce higher levels of both concentric and eccentric torque from the prone (Figure 6.11) than supine (Figure 6.10) position, and both the supine and prone positions more closely simulate the length-tension relationship of these muscles during walking and running than does the seated position (Worrell, Denegar, Armstrong, & Perrin, 1990).

Tables 6.6 and 6.7 present gravity-corrected and non-gravity-corrected normative data for the knee extensor and flexor muscle groups for a variety of

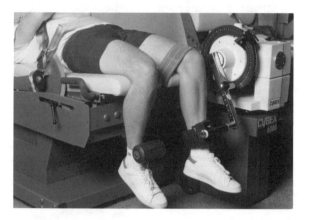

Figure 6.10   Test and exercise position for the knee extensor and flexor muscles while supine. This test position places the rectus femoris in a lengthened position and the hamstring muscles in a shortened position.

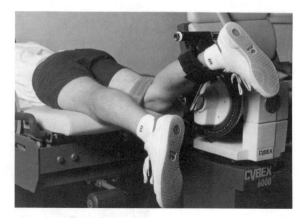

Figure 6.11   Test and exercise position for the knee extensor and flexor muscles while prone. This position approximates the length-tension relationship of the quadriceps and hamstring muscle groups when walking and running.

nondisabled and athletic populations ranging from prepubescents to adults. Regardless of age or activity, the bilateral relationships of the quadriceps and hamstring muscle groups tend to be within 5% to 10% of each other. Moreover, these relationships appear to be essentially the same for both concentric and eccentric values, although eccentric strength is greater than concentric strength for both the quadriceps and hamstring muscle groups. Isokinetic strength of the knee extensor and flexor muscle groups is also frequently reported relative to body weight. Table 6.8 presents strength of the quadriceps and hamstring muscle groups normalized to body weight in a variety of populations.

Normative values for the hamstring/quadriceps reciprocal muscle group ratio are presented in Table 6.9. In general, the hamstring muscle group has been shown to produce about 60% of the torque values generated by the quadriceps muscles at slow isokinetic test velocities. Particularly noteworthy is that test velocity affects the hamstring/quadriceps reciprocal muscle group ratio. Increases in test velocity appear to reduce quadriceps torque to a greater degree than torque of the hamstring muscle group. The hamstring muscle group thus produces a greater percentage of the torque values generated by the quadriceps muscles as test velocity increases, although gravity correction appears to reduce this effect.

Note carefully the presence or absence of a gravity correction procedure when using the normative data from Tables 6.6, 6.7, 6.8, and 6.9. In Tables 6.8 and 6.9, the designation (GC) is included where a gravity correction procedure was mentioned in the data-collection protocol or was confirmed through personal correspondence. As discussed in chapter 3, gravity correction will add to the torque produced by a muscle group contracting against the effect of gravity and will subtract from the muscle group assisted by gravity. If a gravity correction procedure is appropriately employed, the quadriceps torque will be higher and the hamstring torque lower than if a correction procedure has not been used. The comparison of gravity-corrected and noncorrected values by Appen and Duncan (1986), Barr and Duncan (1988), and Fillyaw et al. (1986) in Table 6.6 illustrates this effect. Gravity correction will also influence the changes in the hamstring/quadriceps reciprocal muscle group ratio that occur with increases in test velocity. The gravity-corrected and uncorrected ratios reported by Appen and Duncan (1986) illustrate this effect (Table 6.9). The uncorrected ratios at test velocities of 60, 180, 240, and 300 deg/s were .64, .79, .84, and .84, respectively, while the corrected ratios were .54, .60, .61, and .60, respectively. This observation underscores the importance of noting the presence or absence of a gravity correction procedure when interpreting normative values for the quadriceps and hamstring muscle groups. You should also always employ a gravity correction procedure when assessing the hamstring and quadriceps muscle groups (and any other muscle groups assessed in a gravity-dependent position).

Table 6.10 presents isokinetic strength values for the quadriceps and hamstring muscle groups for populations who have experienced either ligamentous or meniscal pathology of the knee joint. This information should help clinicians establish reasonable bilateral and reciprocal muscle group target values for the rehabilitation of similar injuries. I suggest you review these studies for details pertaining to the length of convalescence, the exact nature of injury and disability, and the relationship between strength and functional status of these patients.

Tibial Internal and External Rotation

Although isokinetic assessment of tibial rotation is somewhat difficult, internal (inward) and external (outward) rotation of the tibia are nonetheless essential to the normal biomechanics of the knee joint (Figure 6.12). Indeed, injury to the anterior cruciate ligament often results in excessive amounts of tibial rotation and is one of the more debilitating injuries that can be experienced by an athlete. Internal tibial rotation is accomplished by the muscles of the pes anserine group (semitendinosus, sartorius, and gracilis) and the popliteus muscle. The popliteus is especially important in initiating flexion by inwardly rotating, or "unlocking," the knee from the terminally extended position (Rasch & Burke, 1978). Outward rotation of the tibia is accomplished primarily by contraction of the biceps femoris muscle. Figure 6.13 illustrates a recommended position for assessing strength of the tibial rotator muscles. Rotation of the tibia with the knee extended beyond approximately 45 deg will be accompanied by inward and outward rotation of the femur. Isolation of tibial rotation is best accomplished by flexing the knee to 90 deg and stabilizing the thigh during assessment. Also, the foot should be immobilized as much as possible to eliminate concomitant pronation and supination of the ankle and foot during assessment of tibial rotation.

There are few reports of isokinetic strength of the tibial rotators in the scientific literature. Table 6.11 presents peak torque values for the internal

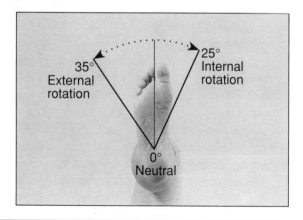

Figure 6.12 Tibial internal and external rotation range of motion.

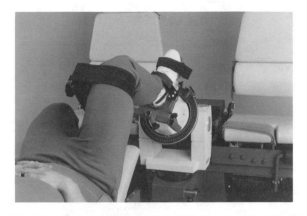

Figure 6.13   Test and exercise position for the tibial internal and external rotator muscles with knee flexed to 90 deg.

and external rotator muscle groups in nondisabled subjects. In general, little difference is seen in the internal or external rotation values between contralateral limbs. Also, very few differences exist between the internal and external rotators within each limb, although strength of the external rotators tends to be slightly but consistently higher than the values for internal rotation.

Patellofemoral Joint Forces

A healthy and efficient patellofemoral articulation is essential to normal biomechanics of the knee joint. Patellofemoral joint pain limits the quadriceps muscle group's ability to extend the knee joint. Isokinetic exercise at slow angular velocities and through extremes of knee flexion has been thought to exacerbate the symptoms associated with patellofemoral dysfunction. Many clinicians therefore consider slow velocity, full range of motion isokinetic exercise as contraindicated for patients experiencing patellofemoral pain. Kaufman et al. (1991) used a mathematical model to calculate the magnitude of patellofemoral compression force during flexion and extension of the knee at test velocities of 60 and 180 deg/s. Patellofemoral compressive forces were found to be low at knee flexion angles less than 20 deg and highest at 70 to 75 deg of knee flexion. Indeed, the maximum compression force was 5.1 times body weight (BW) at 60 deg/s and slightly lower (4.9 × BW) at 180 deg/s. Figures 6.14 and 6.15 illustrate patellofemoral forces during isokinetic exercise from 0 to 100 deg of knee flexion at 60 and 180 deg/s. The clinical implication is that isokinetic exercise beyond 20 deg of knee flexion should be avoided in patients experiencing patellofemoral joint pain. These findings also suggest that patellofemoral joint forces are more related to knee joint position than to exercise velocity. That is, little difference was found in patellofemoral joint forces between the 60 and 180 deg/s test

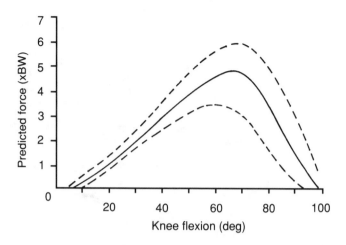

Figure 6.14 Patellofemoral forces during isokinetic exercise at 60 deg/s. All forces have been normalized with respect to the subject's body weight. Solid line is average for five subjects. Dashed line indicates ±1 SD.

From "Dynamic Joint Forces During Knee Isokinetic Exercise" by K.R. Kaufman, K-N An, W.J. Litchy, B.F. Morrey, and E.Y.S. Chao, 1991, *American Journal of Sports Medicine,* **19**(3), p. 310. Copyright 1991 by American Orthopaedic Society for Sports Medicine. Reprinted by permission.

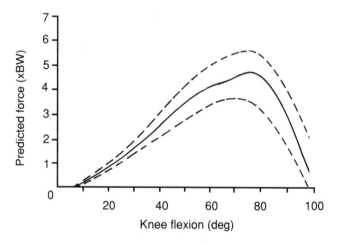

Figure 6.15 Patellofemoral forces during isokinetic exercise at 180 deg/s. All forces have been normalized with respect to the subject's body weight. Solid line is average for five subjects. Dashed line indicates ±1 SD.

From "Dynamic Joint Forces During Knee Isokinetic Exercise" by K.R. Kaufman, K-N An, W.J. Litchy, B.F. Morrey, and E.Y.S. Chao, 1991, *American Journal of Sports Medicine,* **19**(3), p. 311. Copyright 1991 by American Orthopaedic Society for Sports Medicine. Reprinted by permission.

velocity. Additional research needs to examine these patellofemoral forces at exercise velocities that exceed 180 deg/s.

Tibiofemoral Joint Forces

The compressive and shear forces produced at the knee joint during isokinetic exercise should be considered when a rehabilitation program is prescribed. Kaufman et al. (1991) used a triaxial electrogoniometer affixed to the leg to determine the maximum tibiofemoral joint compressive forces during isokinetic exercise at 60 and 180 deg/s. During knee extension, the peak force was 4.0 × BW at 60 deg/s, and was slightly less (3.8 × BW) at 180 deg/s. Patients who have been in a non-weight-bearing state for an extended period of time experience softening of the articular cartilage of the femoral and tibial joint surfaces. The joint compressive forces associated with isokinetic exercise or assessment preclude these patients from this form of resistance therapy until after a gradual period of weight-bearing activity has been completed.

Isokinetic exercise also produces an anterior tibiofemoral joint shear force during extension of the knee. Contraction of the quadriceps muscle group with placement of the resistance pad of the lever arm at the distal tibia tends to force the proximal end of the tibia anteriorly with respect to the distal femur (Nisell, Ericson, Nemeth, & Ekholm, 1989). This force, approximately 0.2 to 0.3 × BW (Kaufman et al., 1991), acts primarily at 25 deg of knee flexion. The anterior cruciate ligament is responsible for checking anterior translation of the tibia on the femur. Take care when providing isokinetic resistance during knee extension in patients experiencing insufficiency or early reconstruction of the anterior cruciate ligament.

The magnitude of anterior shear force is significantly reduced when the resistance pad of the dynamometer is moved closer to the proximal end of the tibia (Nisell et al., 1989). Proximal placement of the resistance pad is recommended to reduce anterior shear of the tibia and thus the amount of stress on the anterior cruciate ligament (Figure 6.16) during knee extension. As the anterior cruciate ligament–insufficient or reconstructed patient progresses through rehabilitation, the resistance pad may be moved distally along the tibia in gradual increments. Proximal placement of the resistance pad should not be used to exercise the hamstring muscle group as it may actually exacerbate the anterior tibial translation during knee flexion. Research is needed to confirm this clinical impression.

Dual-pad resistance devices are commercially available to reduce the anterior shear at the proximal tibia during knee extension exercises (Figure 6.17). A device similar to the one shown in Figure 6.17 (Johnson, 1982) has been shown to be effective in providing resistance to the quadriceps muscle group (Timm, 1986) and in reducing anterior translation of the proximal tibia (Lavin & Gross, 1990).

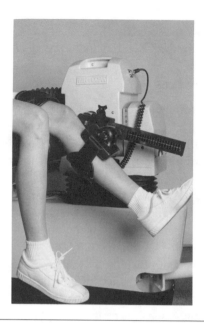

Figure 6.16 Resistance pad placed proximally on tibia to reduce anterior shear of proximal tibia during resisted knee extension.

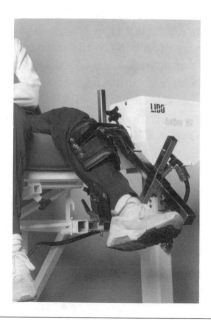

Figure 6.17 Dual resistance pad device designed to reduce anterior shear of proximal tibia during resisted knee extension.

"Closed-Kinetic-Chain" Exercise and Assessment

Lower extremity rehabilitation protocols should include strength training from a weight-bearing or foot-fixed ("closed-kinetic-chain") position. Quantification of human muscular performance is an important component of any rehabilitation program. However, the transferability of isokinetic exercise and assessment from a non-weight-bearing state ("open-kinetic-chain") to the weight-bearing demands of many industrial and athletic activities is questionable. Many isokinetic dynamometers can be used to exercise the major muscle groups of the lower extremity from a foot-fixed (closed-kinetic-chain) position (Engle, 1983; Levine, Klein, & Morrissey, 1991). Figure 6.18, a and b illustrates use of an isokinetic dynamometer as a closed-kinetic-chain exercise device. I advise clinicians to incorporate a variety of weight-bearing functional activities into all lower extremity rehabilitation protocols (Lephart, Perrin, Minger, & Fu, 1991).

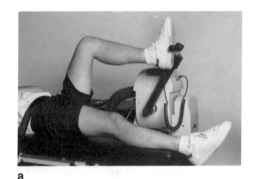
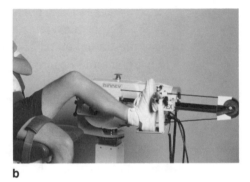

a   b

Figure 6.18   Use of an isokinetic dynamometer for "closed-kinetic-chain" exercise of the knee and hip (a and b).

THE ANKLE JOINT

Movements at the ankle and foot occur at several articulations, which renders the biomechanics of this region quite complicated. This multijoint system is comprised of the talocrural (talus and tibia), subtalar (talus and calcaneus), and transverse tarsal (talonavicular and calcaneocuboid) articulations. For our purposes of isokinetic exercise and assessment, I'll now discuss ankle plantar flexion and dorsiflexion and inversion and eversion.

Ankle Plantar Flexion and Dorsiflexion

Ankle plantar flexion and dorsiflexion occur primarily at the talocrural joint (Figure 6.19, a and b). In general, any muscles passing posterior to the axis of rotation of the malleoli must contribute to plantar flexion of the ankle.

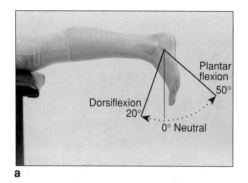
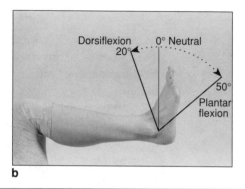

Figure 6.19   Ankle plantar flexion and dorsiflexion range of motion with the knee extended (a) and flexed to 90 deg (b).

In contrast, any muscles passing anterior to this axis of rotation must produce or contribute to ankle dorsiflexion. Ankle plantar flexion is produced primarily by the gastrocnemius and soleus muscles of the triceps sursae complex (see illustration on p. 72). Of these two muscles, only the gastrocnemius is a two-joint muscle, crossing the knee and ankle joints. Isokinetic assessment and exercise of plantar flexion with the knee in the 0 deg extended position will tend to recruit the gastrocnemius muscle to a greater degree, while flexion of the knee to 90 deg will shorten the gastrocnemius and permit greater isolation of the soleus muscle (Figure 6.19, a and b). Plantar flexion strength tends to be greater when assessed with the knee in the 0 deg extended position than when the knee is at 90 deg of flexion (Fugl-Meyer, 1981). Dorsiflexion of the ankle is produced primarily by the tibialis anterior, extensor digitorum longus, and peroneus tertius muscles. Each of these muscles originates from the tibia or fibula and thus are one-joint muscles with respect to their action at the ankle joint. However, even though these muscles do not cross the knee joint, strength of the dorsiflexors tends to be greater when assessment occurs with the knee in the 90 deg flexed position than the 0 deg extended position (Fugl-Meyer, 1981).

Figures 6.20 and 6.21 illustrate common positions for assessment and exercise of the ankle plantar flexor and dorsiflexor muscles. Because optimal strength is produced by the plantar flexors with the knee at 0 deg of extension and the dorsiflexors with the knee at 90 deg of flexion, these positions are recommended for assessment of peak torque of these muscle groups. However, isokinetic exercise should occur with the knee both flexed and extended to ensure isolation of all anterior and posterior muscles of the leg.

Table 6.12 presents normative data for the ankle plantar flexor and dorsiflexor muscles, and Table 6.13 presents the dorsiflexion/plantar flexion reciprocal muscle group ratios. Unless noted otherwise, these values were obtained with the

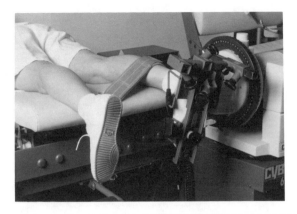

Figure 6.20   Test and exercise position for the ankle plantar flexor and dorsiflexor muscles with knee extended to isolate the gastrocnemius muscle.

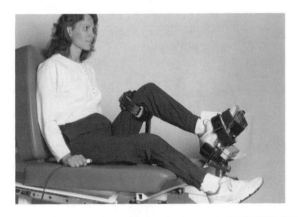

Figure 6.21   Test and exercise position for the ankle plantar flexor and dorsiflexor muscles with knee flexed to isolate the soleus muscle.

knee in the 0 deg extended position. It is clear from Table 6.13 that the plantar flexor muscles produce substantially more torque than the dorsiflexor muscle group. Indeed, for most populations the dorsiflexors produce 30% to 40% of the torque values generated by the plantar flexor muscles. This significant discrepancy in the dorsiflexion/plantar flexion reciprocal muscle group ratio might be partly responsible for the high incidence of anterior leg pain in athletes.

Ankle Inversion and Eversion

Inversion and eversion of the ankle occur through the combined movements of the subtalar, talonavicular, and calcaneocuboid joints (Figure 6.22). In general, any muscle that crosses the ankle to the medial side of the midline of the foot produces inversion, and any muscle that passes lateral to the

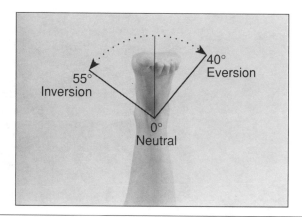

Figure 6.22   Ankle inversion and eversion range of motion.

midline of the foot produces eversion. The primary invertors are the tibialis anterior and tibialis posterior muscles, and the primary evertors include the extensor digitorum longus and the peroneus longus, brevis, and tertius muscles. All of the primary invertors and evertors of the ankle originate from the tibia or fibula and thus do not cross the knee joint. However, changes in position of the knee influence assessment of ankle inversion and eversion peak torque. For example, inversion and eversion strength tend to be stronger with the knee in the flexed position—probably because the medial and lateral hamstring muscles produce concomitant tibial internal and external rotation during assessment of ankle inversion and eversion, respectively (Lentell, Cashman, Shiomoto, & Spry, 1988). So, although peak torque will be less, isolation of the ankle invertors and evertors is best accomplished with the knee in 0 deg of extension (Figure 6.23).

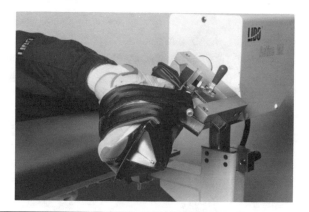

Figure 6.23   Test and exercise position for the ankle invertor and evertor muscles with knee extended.

The position of the foot in dorsiflexion, neutral, or plantar flexion also has an influence on assessment of ankle inversion and eversion peak torque. In general, greater inversion and eversion torque is produced as the foot is moved from the dorsiflexed to the plantar flexed position (Cawthorn, Cummings, Walker, & Donatelli, 1991). Apparently, 10 deg of plantar flexion optimizes the actin-myosin coupling process for the muscles, primarily producing inversion and eversion of the ankle. Figure 6.24 illustrates an additional position for exercise and assessment of the ankle invertor and evertor muscles.

Table 6.14 presents normative data for the ankle invertor and evertor muscle groups, and Table 6.15 presents the limited normative data for the eversion/inversion reciprocal muscle group ratios. In general, we see little difference between right and left sides for both the invertor and evertor muscles. Also, the reciprocal muscle group ratio indicates that the invertor muscles produce only slightly more torque than that generated by the evertor muscles.

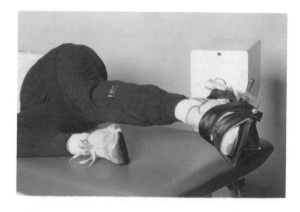

Figure 6.24   Test and exercise position for the ankle invertor and evertor muscles with knee flexed to 45 deg.

RELIABILITY OF LOWER EXTREMITY ASSESSMENT

The reliability of assessing isokinetic strength of the quadriceps and hamstring muscle groups has been adequately established in the literature. Reliability is quite high across a spectrum of test velocities for both muscle groups. As with the upper extremity, reliability of eccentric torque measurement tends to be slightly less than assessment of concentric torque.

Very few studies have examined the reliability of isokinetic assessment of the hip and ankle musculature. And virtually none have established the reliability of assessing eccentric torque of these muscle groups. More research is needed to establish the reliability of concentric and eccentric isokinetic assessment of the muscles acting on both the hip and ankle joints.

Table 6.16 summarizes several published reports of reliability of assessing the knee extensor and flexor muscles, as well as the limited studies of hip and ankle assessment. As with the upper extremity, I advise you to note the statistical technique, subject population, test position, and isokinetic instrumentation used when drawing conclusions about the reliability of isokinetic assessment from Table 6.16.

Table 6.1
Normative Values of Hip Flexion and Extension Peak Torque (in ft-lb)

Study and population	Sex	Age	Dominant flexion	Nondominant flexion	Dominant extension	Nondominant extension
			30 deg/s			
Smith et al. (1981) Professional and elite amateur ice hockey players	M	24	128.3		204.0	
Smith et al. (1982) Canadian Olympic hockey team	M	22	124.7		202.8	
Poulmedis (1985) Elite soccer players	M	28	132.0		198.4	
Nicholas et al. (1989) Nondisabled	M	20-30	77.0		98.0	
	F	20-30	55.0		83.0	
Alexander (1990) Elite sprinters (Dom = average of left and right limb scores)	M	22	171.8		230.1	
		(E)	192.5		254.4	
	F	20	120.2		156.4	
		(E)	137.9		191.8	
			60 deg/s			
Tippett (1986) College baseball pitchers (Dom = stance extremity; NDom= kick extremity)	M	20	105.0	118.0	200.0	191.0
			90 deg/s			
Poulmedis (1985) Elite soccer players	M	28	95.1		153.4	
			180 deg/s			
Smith et al. (1981) Professional and elite amateur ice hockey players	M	24	83.9		149.8	
Smith et al. (1982) Canadian Olympic hockey team	M	22	79.7		145.8	
Poulmedis (1985) Elite soccer players	M	28	70.1		119.5	

(continued)

Table 6.1 *(continued)*

Study and population	Sex	Age	Dominant flexion	Nondominant flexion	Dominant extension	Nondominant extension
Alexander (1990)						
Elite sprinters (Dom =	M	22	145.3		230.1	
average of left and right		(E)	177.7		268.5	
limb scores)	F	20	107.0		171.1	
		(E)	129.8		205.0	
			240 deg/s			
Tippett (1986)						
College baseball pitchers	M	20	70.0	69.0	173.0	174.0
(Dom = stance extremity;						
NDom = kick extremity)						

Note. Dom—dominant; NDom—nondominant; E—eccentric.

Table 6.2
Normative Values of Hip Flexion/Extension Reciprocal Muscle Group Ratios (Percent)

Study and population	Sex	Age	Dominant flexion/extension ratio	Nondominant flexion/extension ratio
30 deg/s				
Smith et al. (1981)				
Professional and elite amateur ice hockey players	M	24	.64	
Poulmedis (1985)				
Elite soccer players	M	28	.66	
Alexander (1990)				
Elite sprinters (Dom = average of left and right limb scores)	M	22	.74	
		(E)	.75	
	F	20	.79	
		(E)	.74	
180 deg/s				
Smith et al. (1981)				
Professional and elite amateur ice hockey players	M	24	.59	
Alexander (1990)				
Elite sprinters (Dom = average of left and right limb scores)	M	22	.59	
		(E)	.66	
	F	20	.65	
		(E)	.65	

Note. Dom—dominant; E—eccentric.

Table 6.3
Normative Values of Hip Abduction and Adduction Peak Torque (in ft-lb)

Study and population	Sex	Age	Dominant abduction	Nondominant abduction	Dominant adduction	Nondominant adduction
30 deg/s						
Poulmedis (1985)						
Elite soccer players	M	28	87.8		118.0	
Tippett (1986)						
College baseball pitchers (Dom = stance extremity; NDom = kick extremity)	M	20	80.0	87.0	104.0	107.0
60 deg/s						
Donatelli et al. (1991)						
Nondisabled (Dom =	F	26	42.6		108.2	
average of right and	M	26	63.8		152.6	
left sides)						
90 deg/s						
Poulmedis (1985)						
Elite soccer players	M	28	64.9		101.0	
180 deg/s						
Poulmedis (1985)						
Elite soccer players	M	28	48.7		80.4	
Tippett (1986)						
College baseball pitchers (Dom = stance extremity; NDom = kick extremity)	M	20	48.0	44.0	96.0	97.0

Note. Dom—dominant; NDom—nondominant.

Table 6.4
Normative Values of Hip Abduction/Adduction Reciprocal Muscle Group Ratios (Percent)

Study and population	Sex	Age	Dominant abduction/adduction ratio	Nondominant abduction/adduction ratio
		30 deg/s		
Poulmedis (1985)				
Elite soccer players	M	28	.74	
		60 deg/s		
Donatelli et al. (1991)				
Nondisabled (Dom = average	F	26	.41	
of right and left sides)	M	26	.48	

Note. Dom—dominant.

Table 6.5
Normative Values of Hip Internal and External Rotation Peak Torque (in ft-lb)

Study and population	Sex	Age	Dominant internal rotation	Nondominant internal rotation	Dominant external rotation	Nondominant external rotation
Tippett (1986)						
College baseball pitchers						
(Dom = stance extremity;						
NDom = kick extremity)						
30 deg/s	M	20	30.0	30.0	25.0	26.0
180 deg/s	M	20	17.0	16.0	16.0	13.0

Note. Dom—dominant; NDom—nondominant.

Table 6.6
Gravity-Corrected Normative Values of Knee Extension and Flexion Peak Torque (in ft-lb)

Study and population	Sex	Age	Dominant extension	Nondominant extension	Dominant flexion	Nondominant flexion
30 deg/s						
Poulmedis (1985)						
Elite soccer players	M	28	182.1		107.7	
60 deg/s						
Schlinkman (1984)						
High school football players	M	15-17	173.0		94.0	
Fillyaw et al. (1986)						
University soccer players	F	19	87.0		46.7	
			82.5 (NGC)		55.4 (NGC)	
Appen & Duncan (1986)						
College track athletes	M	18-21	149.0 (NGC)		95.0 (NGC)	
			156.0		83.0	
Worrell et al. (1990)						
University lacrosse players	F	19			47.1*	46.7*
(reported as average torque)		(E)			58.6*	60.0*
					29.8+	29.7+
		(E)			40.9+	40.9+
Ghena et al. (1991)						
Athletes	M	20	191.4		104.9	
		(E)	189.8		122.5	
90 deg/s						
Poulmedis (1985)						
Elite soccer players	M	28	140.9		92.2	
Barr & Duncan (1988)						
Nondisabled (supine)	M and F	27				45.6
						60.8 (NGC)
Nondisabled (prone)	M and F	27				70.0
						45.0 (NGC)
120 deg/s						
Ghena et al. (1991)						
Athletes	M	20	161.7		92.7	
		(E)	192.0		123.8	

Table 6.6 *(continued)*

Study and population	Sex	Age	Dominant extension	Nondominant extension	Dominant flexion	Nondominant flexion
			180 deg/s			
Poulmedis (1985)						
Elite soccer players	M	28	92.9		68.6	
Appen & Duncan (1986)						
College track athletes	M	18-21	94.0 (NGC)		73.0 (NGC)	
			105.0		63.0	
			240 deg/s			
Schlinkman (1984)						
High school football players	M	15-17	98.0		65.0	
Fillyaw et al. (1986)						
University soccer players	F	19	49.6		25.3	
			42.5 (NGC)		33.5 (NGC)	
Appen & Duncan (1986)						
College track athletes	M	18-21	77.0 (NGC)		63.0 (NGC)	
			89.0		54.0	
			300 deg/s			
Schlinkman (1984)						
High school football players	M	15-17	83.0		56.0	
Appen & Duncan (1986)						
College track athletes	M	18-21	67.0 (NGC)		57.0 (NGC)	
			78.0		48.0	
Klopfer & Greij (1988)						
Nondisabled (Dom =	F	28	36.5		36.9	
average of right and	M	27	76.8		56.0	
left sides)						
Ghena et al. (1991)						
Athletes	M	20	107.5		65.2	
			330 deg/s			
Klopfer & Greij (1988)						
Nondisabled (Dom =	F	28	35.1		37.8	
average of right and	M	27	74.1		62.3	
left sides)						

(continued)

Table 6.6 *(continued)*

Study and population	Sex	Age	Dominant extension	Nondominant extension	Dominant flexion	Nondominant flexion
			360 deg/s			
Klopfer & Greij (1988)						
Nondisabled (Dom =	F	28	33.8		37.8	
average of right and	M	27	73.2		60.6	
left sides)						
			400 deg/s			
Klopfer & Greij (1988)						
Nondisabled (Dom =	F	28	34.0		38.8	
average of right and	M	27	68.9		58.9	
left sides)						
			450 deg/s			
Klopfer & Greij (1988)						
Nondisabled (Dom =	F	28	34.2		37.0	
average of right and	M	27	69.9		67.9	
left sides)						
Ghena et al. (1991)						
Athletes	M	20	83.4		67.6	

Note. NGC—no gravity correction procedure used; Dom—dominant; E—eccentric; *—prone; [+]—supine.

Table 6.7

Non-Gravity-Corrected Normative Values of Knee Extension and Flexion Peak Torque (in ft-lb)

Study and population	Sex	Age	Dominant extension	Nondominant extension	Dominant flexion	Nondominant flexion
			30 deg/s			
Gilliam et al. (1979)						
Active children (Dom =	M	7-13	52.3		30.9	
average of right and	F	7-13	53.9		31.9	
left sides adjusted						
[ANCOVA] for age)						
Haymes & Dickinson (1980)						
Alpine ski racers	F	19	139.5			
	M	22	191.5			
Smith et al. (1981)						
Professional and elite	M	24	207.3		128.0	
amateur ice hockey players						
Smith et al. (1982)						
Canadian Olympic hockey	M	22	215.5		126.6	
team						
Morris et al. (1983)						
College middle-distance	M	20	139.2		87.0	
and distance runners						
Costain & Williams (1984)						
Adolescent soccer players	F	15-17	132.0	129.0	80.4	79.1
Weltman et al. (1988)						
Prepubertal boys (values	M	6-11	26.7	29.1	41.9	45.0
expressed as mean work						
output)						
Hanten & Ramberg (1988)						
Nondisabled	F	25	133.0			
		(E)	168.9			
Hageman et al. (1988)						
Nondisabled	M	21-33	194.6	183.5	106.9	113.7
		(E)	205.4	188.9	127.7	132.2
	F	21-33	108.9	107.6	63.6	65.3
		(E)	120.6	120.6	76.0	76.6
Westing et al. (1988)						
Well-trained physical	M	25		174.8		
education students		(E)		211.7		
(NDom = left side						
values)						

(continued)

Table 6.7 *(continued)*

Study and population	Sex	Age	Dominant extension	Nondominant extension	Dominant flexion	Nondominant flexion
Colliander & Tesch (1989)						
Physically active	F	27	197.7		115.1	
nondisabled		(E)	267.7		124.6	
	M	27	311.2		178.5	
		(E)	387.2		194.0	
Alexander (1990)						
Elite sprinters (Dom =	M	22	196.9		124.6	
average of left and right		(E)	205.8		131.3	
limb scores)	F	20	126.1		81.9	
		(E)	135.0		87.8	
Knapik et al. (1991)						
Collegiate athletes	F	19	115.1	109.9	68.6	70.1
			60 deg/s			
Wyatt & Edwards (1981)						
Nondisabled	M	29	137.0	132.0	98.0	93.0
	F	28	80.0	79.0	57.0	55.0
Morris et al. (1983)						
College middle-distance	M	20	132.6		86.7	
and distance runners						
Thomas (1984)						
Nondisabled (values for	F	35		65.5		38.2
left leg)						
Holmes & Alderink (1984)						
High school students	F	16	100.2	99.7	55.2	55.7
	M	17	151.0	146.1	86.6	86.3
Tabin et al. (1985)						
Prepubescent (PreP) and	F	PreP	71.9			
postpubescent (PstP)	M	PreP	67.2			
athletes (values expressed	F	PstP	81.2			
as peak torque/lean	M	PstP	88.8			
body weight)						
DiBrezzo et al. (1985)						
Nondisabled (seated with	F	21	96.5		51.9	
backrest at 20 deg from						
vertical)						

Table 6.7 *(continued)*

Study and population	Sex	Age	Dominant extension	Nondominant extension	Dominant flexion	Nondominant flexion
60 deg/s						
Berg et al. (1985) College basketball players (Dom = right side values; NDom = left side values)	F	20	121.8	116.9	76.2	77.8
Tippett (1986) College baseball pitchers (Dom = stance extremity; NDom = kick extremity)	M	20	194.0	190.0	123.0	122.0
Hanten & Ramberg (1988) Nondisabled	F	25 (E)	124.3 170.8			
Chmelar et al. (1988) Ballet and modern dancers (values expressed as peak torque/body weight)	F	25	75.9		46.2	
Nicholas et al. (1989) Nondisabled	M F	20-30 20-30	109.0 76.0		75.0 42.0	
Lucca & Kline (1989) Nondisabled	F M	21 21	96.7 154.2	97.4 162.7	62.5 98.2	63.5 93.5
90 deg/s						
Stafford & Grana (1984) College football players	M	20	161.1	157.6	107.1	107.2
Weltman et al. (1988) Prepubertal boys (values expressed as mean work output)	M	6-11	22.4	24.9	35.0	36.9
Hanten & Ramberg (1988) Nondisabled	F	25 (E)	114.2 173.9			
Chmelar et al. (1988) Ballet and modern dancers (values expressed as peak torque/body weight)	F	25	66.5		44.4	

(continued)

Table 6.7 *(continued)*

Study and population	Sex	Age	Dominant extension	Nondominant extension	Dominant flexion	Nondominant flexion
Colliander & Tesch (1989)						
Physically active	F	27	167.4		102.5	
nondisabled		(E)	290.6		138.7	
	M	27	267.7		165.9	
		(E)	372.4		199.9	
			120 deg/s			
Gilliam et al. (1979)						
Active children (Dom =	M	7-13	37.5		27.6	
average of right and left	F	7-13	36.9		27.2	
sides adjusted [ANCOVA]						
for age)						
Berg et al. (1985)						
College basketball players	F	20	97.9	96.6	66.1	68.8
(Dom = right side values;						
NDom = left side values)						
Hanten & Ramberg (1988)						
Nondisabled	F	25	101.4			
		(E)	158.9			
Westing et al. (1988)						
Well-trained physical	M	25		137.2		
education students		(E)		212.4		
(NDom = left side values)						
			150 deg/s			
Hanten & Ramberg (1988)						
Nondisabled	F	25	94.8			
		(E)	167.9			
Colliander & Tesch (1989)						
Physically active	F	27	135.7		95.1	
nondisabled		(E)	273.6		142.3	
	M	27	227.2		154.1	
		(E)	358.4		201.3	

Table 6.7 *(continued)*

Study and population	Sex	Age	Dominant extension	Nondominant extension	Dominant flexion	Nondominant flexion
			180 deg/s			
Haymes & Dickinson (1980)						
Alpine ski racers	F	19	77.4			
	M	22	123.6			
Wyatt & Edwards (1981)						
Nondisabled	M	29	98.0	96.0	77.0	74.0
	F	28	58.0	56.0	46.0	45.0
Smith et al. (1981)						
Professional and elite amateur ice hockey players	M	24	107.2		86.4	
Smith et al. (1982)						
Canadian Olympic hockey team	M	22	110.2		83.5	
Morris et al. (1983)						
College middle-distance and distance runners	M	20	88.2		66.1	
Stafford & Grana (1984)						
College football players	M	20	122.1	116.6	88.2	87.0
Costain & Williams (1984)						
Adolescent soccer players	F	15-17	62.1	61.6	48.8	47.2
Holmes & Alderink (1984)						
High school students	F	16	56.7	56.9	38.5	38.0
	M	17	88.1	84.9	61.9	60.7
Housh et al. (1984)						
Adolescent track and field athletes	F	16	79.0		58.8	
Berg et al. (1985)						
College basketball players (Dom = right side values; NDom = left side values)	F	20	78.7	79.8	56.3	57.7
Hanten & Ramberg (1988)						
Nondisabled	F	25	86.4			
		(E)	167.2			
Hageman et al. (1988)						
Nondisabled	M	21-33	135.3	123.8	104.0	113.6
		(E)	198.0	188.8	130.8	137.2
	F	21-33	72.2	72.9	60.3	65.3
		(E)	123.0	117.9	84.5	83.7

(continued)

Table 6.7 *(continued)*

Study and population	Sex	Age	Dominant extension	Nondominant extension	Dominant flexion	Nondominant flexion
Chmelar et al. (1988)						
Ballet and modern dancers (values expressed as peak torque/body weight)	F	25	47.8		37.8	
Nicholas et al. (1989)						
Nondisabled	M	20-30	70.0		50.0	
	F	20-30	44.0		24.0	
Lucca & Kline (1989)						
Nondisabled	F	21	64.4	66.0	49.3	49.8
	M	21	113.6	111.1	75.0	75.1
Knapik et al. (1991)						
Collegiate athletes	F	19	66.4	66.4	50.9	50.9
200 deg/s						
Hanten & Ramberg (1988)						
Nondisabled	F	25	83.9			
		(E)	165.0			
230 deg/s						
Alexander (1990)						
Elite sprinters (Dom = average of left and right limb scores)	M	22	156.4		122.4	
		(E)	203.6		129.8	
	F	20	93.7		80.0	
		(E)	137.9		95.9	
240 deg/s						
Morris et al. (1983)						
College middle-distance and distance runners	M	20	70.6		57.9	
Thomas (1984)						
Nondisabled (values for left leg)	F	35		23.3		18.7
Berg et al. (1985)						
College basketball players (Dom = right side values; NDom = left side values)	F	20	65.5	65.2	49.7	51.8

Table 6.7 *(continued)*

Study and population	Sex	Age	Dominant extension	Nondominant extension	Dominant flexion	Nondominant flexion
			240 deg/s			

Tippett (1986)
  College baseball pitchers
  (Dom = stance extremity;
  NDom = kick extremity)
	M	20	110.0	114.0	88.0	92.0

Chmelar et al. (1988)
  Ballet and modern dancers
  (values expressed as peak
  torque/body weight)
	F	25	38.1		33.9	

Lucca & Kline (1989) Nondisabled	F	21	54.8	54.8	46.5	44.8
	M	21	95.7	98.0	67.8	70.1
			270 deg/s			

Westing et al. (1988)
  Well-trained physical
  education students
  (NDom = left side values)
	M	25
		(E)
				93.7
				220.5		

			300 deg/s			
Wyatt & Edwards (1981) Nondisabled	M	29	67.0	65.0	55.0	53.0
	F	28	38.0	38.0	32.0	32.0

Morris et al. (1983)
  College middle-distance
  and distance runners
	M	20	59.3		51.4	

Stafford & Grana (1984) College football players	M	20	75.0	70.4	61.4	59.5

Berg et al. (1985)
  College basketball players
  (Dom = right side values;
  NDom = left side values)
	F	20	50.4	50.8	39.7	42.9

Note. Dom—dominant; NDom—nondominant; ANCOVA—analysis of covariance; E—eccentric.

Table 6.8
Normative Values of Knee Extension and Flexion Expressed as a Percentage of Body Weight

Study and population	Sex	Age	Dominant extension	Nondominant extension	Dominant flexion	Nondominant flexion
30 deg/s						
Hageman et al. (1988)						
Nondisabled (values	M	21-33	3.18		1.85	
expressed as Nm/kg		(E)	3.30		2.18	
body weight)	F	21-33	2.48		1.48	
		(E)	2.74		1.75	
Colliander & Tesch (1989)						
Physically active nondis-	F	27	4.78		2.78	
abled (values expressed		(E)	6.47		3.00	
as Nm/kg body weight)	M	27	5.76		3.30	
		(E)	7.17		3.59	
Alexander (1990)						
Elite sprinters (values	M	22	3.65		2.32	
expressed as Nm/kg body		(E)	3.83		2.43	
weight; Dom = average of	F	20	2.95		1.93	
left and right limb scores)		(E)	3.14		2.07	
50 deg/s						
Highgenboten et al. (1988)						
Nondisabled (values	M	15-24	2.98		1.21	
expressed as Nm/kg body		(E)	3.09		1.44	
weight; Dom = average	M	25-34	2.49		1.08	
of right and left sides)		(E)	2.67		1.37	
	F	15-24	2.19		.87	
		(E)	2.37		1.06	
	F	25-34	1.98		.85	
		(E)	2.36		1.11	
60 deg/s						
Schlinkman (1984)						
High school football players	M	15-17	113.0		60.0	
(values expressed as ft-lb/lb						
body weight) (GC)						
Lucca & Kline (1989)						
Nondisabled (values	F	21	75.0	76.0	48.0	50.0
expressed as ft-lb/lb	M	21	93.0	98.0	59.0	56.0
body weight)						

Table 6.8 *(continued)*

Study and population	Sex	Age	Dominant extension	Nondominant extension	Dominant flexion	Nondominant flexion
60 deg/s						
Worrell et al. (1991)						
Athletes (values expressed	M	21	2.95	2.85	1.83	1.81
as Nm/kg body weight) (GC)		(E)	3.14	3.05	1.77	1.75
90 deg/s						
Colliander & Tesch (1989)						
Physically active nondis-	F	27	4.03		2.46	
abled (values expressed as		(E)	7.02		3.32	
Nm/kg body weight)	M	27	4.96		3.06	
		(E)	6.90		3.70	
150 deg/s						
Colliander & Tesch (1989)						
Physically active nondis-	F	27	3.26		2.29	
abled (values expressed as		(E)	6.58		3.41	
Nm/kg body weight)	M	27	4.22		2.84	
		(E)	6.67		3.71	
180 deg/s						
Hageman et al. (1988)						
Nondisabled (values	M	21-33	2.17		1.83	
expressed as Nm/kg		(E)	3.23		2.25	
body weight)	F	21-33	1.66		1.44	
		(E)	2.77		1.93	
Lucca & Kline (1989)						
Nondisabled (values	F	21	50.0	52.0	39.0	39.0
expressed as ft-lb/lb	M	21	68.0	67.0	45.0	45.0
body weight)						
Worrell et al. (1991)						
Athletes (values expressed	M	21	2.35	2.32	1.59	1.64
as Nm/kg body weight) (GC)		(E)	3.50	3.40	2.02	1.98

(continued)

Table 6.8 *(continued)*

Study and population	Sex	Age	Dominant extension	Nondominant extension	Dominant flexion	Nondominant flexion
			230 deg/s			
Alexander (1990)						
Elite sprinters (values ex-	M	22	2.90		2.25	
pressed as Nm/kg body		(E)	3.78		2.41	
weight; Dom = average of	F	20	2.21		1.87	
left and right limb scores)		(E)	3.22		2.24	
			240 deg/s			
Schlinkman (1984)						
High school football	M	15-17	64.0		42.0	
players (values expressed						
as ft-lb/lb body weight) (GC)						
Lucca & Kline (1989)						
Nondisabled (values	F	21	43.0	43.0	36.0	35.0
expressed as ft-lb/lb	M	21	58.0	59.0	41.0	42.0
body weight)						
			300 deg/s			
Schlinkman (1984)						
High school football players	M	15-17	54.0		36.0	
(values expressed as ft-lb/lb						
body weight) (GC)						

Note. E—eccentric; Dom—dominant; GC—gravity correction procedure used.

Table 6.9
Normative Values of Knee Flexion/Extension Reciprocal Muscle Group Ratios (Percent)

Study and population	Sex	Age	Dominant flexion/extension ratio	Nondominant flexion/extension ratio
		15 deg/s		
Figoni et al. (1988)				
Nondisabled (* = hip angle at 5 deg of flexion; + = hip angle at 120 deg of flexion)	M	24	.50* .38 (GC)* .70+ .59 (GC)+	
		30 deg/s		
Gilliam et al. (1979)				
Active children (Dom = average of right and left sides adjusted [ANCOVA] for age)	M	7-13	.61	
	F	7-13	.60	
Smith et al. (1981)				
Professional and elite amateur ice hockey players	M	24	.62	
Costain & Williams (1984)				
Adolescent soccer players	F	15-17	.61	.62
Poulmedis (1985)				
Elite soccer players (GC)	M	28	.60	
Oberg et al. (1986)				
Soccer players (GC)	M	24-26	.61	
Nonsoccer players (GC)	M	21	.57	
Hageman et al. (1988)				
Nondisabled	M	21-33	.55	.62
		(E)	.62	.70
	F	21-33	.59	.62
		(E)	.67	.63
Colliander & Tesch (1989)				
Physically active nondisabled	F	27	.59	
		(E)	.48	
	M	27	.58	
		(E)	.51	
Alexander (1990)				
Elite sprinters (Dom = average of left and right limb scores)	M	22	.64	
		(E)	.63	
	F	20	.65	
		(E)	.66	

(continued)

Table 6.9 *(continued)*

Study and population	Sex	Age	Dominant flexion/extension ratio	Nondominant flexion/extension ratio
		50 deg/s		
Highgenboten et al. (1988)				
Nondisabled (Dom = average	M	15-34	.43	
of right and left sides)		(E)	.51	
	F	15-34	.42	
		(E)	.49	
		60 deg/s		
Holmes & Alderink (1984)				
High school students	F	16	.55	
	M	17	.58	
Schlinkman (1984)				
High school football players (GC)	M	15-17	.54	
Thomas (1984)				
Nondisabled (value for left side)	F	35		.60
Berg et al. (1985)				
College basketball players	F	20	.63	.67
Tabin et al. (1985)				
Prepubescent (PreP) and	F	PreP	.64	
postpubescent (PstP) athletes	M	PreP	.66	
	F	PstP	.62	
	M	PstP	.59	
Fillyaw et al. (1986)				
University soccer players	F	19	.67	
			.54 (GC)	
Appen & Duncan (1986)				
College track athletes	M	18-21	.64	
			.54 (GC)	
Burnie (1987)				
Preadolescents	M	11	.65	.67
Preadolescent gymnasts	F	11	.61	.58
Chmelar et al. (1988)				
Ballet and modern dancers	F	25	.62	
Kannus (1988c)				
Chronic ACL–insufficient subjects	F and M	35	.64	.68
(NDom = ACL–insufficient knee;				
Dom = uninjured knee) (GC)				

Table 6.9 *(continued)*

Study and population	Sex	Age	Dominant flexion/extension ratio	Nondominant flexion/extension ratio
Lucca & Kline (1989)				
Nondisabled	F	21	.66	.67
	M	21	.66	.58
Worrell et al. (1991)				
Healthy athletes and athletes* with	M	21	.65*	.61*
history of hamstring injury (NDom =		(E)	.51*	.52*
hamstring injured extremity or matched			.64	.64
extremity in uninjured subjects; Dom =		(E)	.56	.59
uninjured extremity) (GC)				
90 deg/s				
Colliander & Tesch (1989)				
Physically active nondisabled	F	27	.61	
		(E)	.48	
	M	27	.63	
		(E)	.54	
Stafford & Grana (1984)				
College football players	M	20	.67	.68
Chmelar et al. (1988)				
Ballet and modern dancers	F	25	.67	
Figoni et al. (1988)				
Nondisabled (* = hip angle at 5 deg	M	24	.58*	
of flexion; + = hip angle at 120 deg			.44 (GC)*	
of flexion)			.66+	
			.53 (GC)+	
120 deg/s				
Gilliam et al. (1979)				
Active children (Dom = average of	M	7-13	.75	
right and left sides adjusted	F	7-13	.76	
[ANCOVA] for age)				
Berg et al. (1985)				
College basketball players	F	20	.67	.71
(Dom = right side values;				
NDom = left side values)				
Burnie (1987)				
Preadolescent gymnasts	F	11	.67	.71

(continued)

Table 6.9 *(continued)*

Study and population	Sex	Age	Dominant flexion/extension ratio	Nondominant flexion/extension ratio
		150 deg/s		
Colliander & Tesch (1989)				
Physically active nondisabled	F	27	.70	
		(E)	.53	
	M	27	.69	
		(E)	.57	
		180 deg/s		
Smith et al. (1981)				
Professional and elite amateur ice hockey players	M	24	.81	
Holmes & Alderink (1984)				
High school students	F	16	.68	
	M	17	.70	
Costain & Williams (1984)				
Adolescent soccer players	F	15-17	.79	.77
Stafford & Grana (1984)				
College football players	M	20	.73	.75
Berg et al. (1985)				
College basketball players (Dom = right side values; NDom = left side values)	F	20	.72	.74
Appen & Duncan (1986)				
College track athletes	M	18-21	.79	
			.60 (GC)	
Oberg et al. (1986)				
Soccer players (GC)	M	24-26	.75	
Nonsoccer players (GC)	M	21	.62	
Hageman et al. (1988)				
Nondisabled	M	21-33	.76	.88
		(E)	.67	.73
	F	21-33	.84	.87
		(E)	.70	.70
Chmelar et al. (1988)				
Ballet and modern dancers	F	25	.80	

Table 6.9 *(continued)*

Study and population	Sex	Age	Dominant flexion/extension ratio	Nondominant flexion/extension ratio
180 deg/s				
Kannus (1988c)				
Chronic ACL–insufficient subjects (NDom = ACL–insufficient knee; Dom = uninjured knee) (GC)	F and M	35	.78	.88
Lucca & Kline (1989)				
Nondisabled	F	21	.78	.76
	M	21	.66	.69
Alexander (1990)				
Elite sprinters (Dom = average of left and right limb scores)	M	22 (E)	.77 .64	
	F	20 (E)	.85 .69	
Worrell et al. (1991)				
Healthy athletes and athletes* with history of hamstring injury (NDom = hamstring injured extremity or matched extremity in uninjured subjects; Dom = uninjured extremity) (GC)	M	21 (E)	.71* .55* .71 .57	.66* .55* .71 .59
240 deg/s				
Schlinkman (1984)				
High school football players (GC)	M	15-17	.66	
Thomas (1984)				
Nondisabled (value for left side)	F	35		.81
Berg et al. (1985)				
College basketball players (Dom = right side values; NDom = left side values)	F	20	.76	.79
Fillyaw et al. (1986)				
University soccer players	F	19	.79 .51 (GC)	
Appen & Duncan (1986)				
College track athletes	M	18-21	.84 .61 (GC)	

(continued)

Table 6.9 *(continued)*

Study and population	Sex	Age	Dominant flexion/extension ratio	Nondominant flexion/extension ratio
Burnie (1987)				
Preadolescents	M	11	.77	.81
Chmelar et al. (1988)				
Ballet and modern dancers	F	25	.90	
Lucca & Kline (1989)				
Nondisabled	F	21	.86	.82
	M	21	.71	.72
300 deg/s				
Schlinkman (1984)				
High school football players (GC)	M	15-17	.67	
Stafford & Grana (1984)				
College football players	M	20	.82	.85
Berg et al. (1985)				
College basketball players (Dom = right side values; NDom = left side values)	F	20	.79	.84
Appen & Duncan (1986)				
College track athletes	M	18-21	.84 .60 (GC)	
Burnie (1987)				
Preadolescent gymnasts	F	11	.91	.98

Note. GC—gravity correction procedure used; Dom—dominant; NDom—nondominant; ANCOVA—analysis of covariance; E—eccentric.

Table 6.10
Values of Knee Extension and Flexion Peak Torque (in ft-lb) on Assessment Following Knee Injury

Study and population	Sex	Age	Uninjured side extension	Chronically injured or postoperative side extension	Uninjured side flexion	Chronically injured or postoperative side flexion
30 deg/s						
Watkins et al. (1983) Patients with history of patellectomy	F and M	29	98.0	45.0	54.0	49.0
60 deg/s						
Campbell & Glenn (1979) Subjects after rehabilitated medial postmeniscectomy	M and F	18-50	113.9	96.1	66.5	58.4
Kannus (1988c) Chronic ACL–insufficient subjects (GC)	F and M	35	123.2	105.5	78.9	70.8
Kannus (1988d) Chronic MCL–injured subjects (GC)	M and F	35	79.7	67.9	47.9	42.0
Kannus & Jarvinen (1989) Chronic ACL–insufficient subjects	M and F	32	122.4	104.0	78.2	70.1
Kannus (1991) Chronic LCL–insufficient subjects (GC)	M and F	35	115.1	110.6	70.8	70.1
120 deg/s						
Morrissey (1987) Subjects with partial meniscectomy	M	17-61	132.0	106.0	99.0	94.0
Harter et al. (1988) ACL–reconstructed subjects (GC)	M and F	24	117.2	100.7	69.0	64.5
Seto et al. (1988) ACL–reconstructed subjects	M and F	32	136.7	121.2*	98.3	96.8*
	M and F	31	126.4	85.4+	98.1	82.0+
Harter et al. (1990) Postoperative ACL– injured subjects (GC)	F	24	92.4	51.3	76.6	47.1
	M	24	133.2	80.4	116.2	75.6

(continued)

Table 6.10 *(continued)*

Study and population	Sex	Age	Uninjured side extension	Chronically injured or postoperative side extension	Ininjured side flexion	Chronically injured or postoperative side flexion
180 deg/s						
Watkins et al. (1983) Patients with history of patellectomy	F and M	29	38.0	22.0	30.0	23.0
Morrissey (1987) Subjects with partial meniscectomy	M	17-61	113.0	92.0	92.0	86.0
Kannus (1988d) Chronic MCL–injured subjects (GC)	M and F	35	45.7	39.1	33.2	25.8
Kannus (1988c) Chronic ACL–insufficient subjects (GC)	F and M	35	69.3	56.1	54.6	47.9
Kannus & Jarvinen (1989) Chronic ACL–insufficient subjects	M and F	32	68.6	55.3	53.8	47.2
Kannus (1991) Chronic LCL–insufficient subjects (GC)	M and F	35	69.3	64.9	49.4	48.7
210 deg/s						
Campbell & Glenn (1979) Subjects after rehabilitated medial post-meniscectomy	M and F	18-50	63.5	54.5	46.4	40.3
240 deg/s						
Morrissey (1987) Subjects with partial meniscectomy	M	17-61	98.0	78.0	77.0	73.0
Seto et al. (1988) ACL–reconstructed subjects	M and F M and F	32 31	89.4 81.7	73.8* 48.5[+]	68.1 62.2	62.7* 53.0[+]

Note. GC—gravity correction procedure used; ACL—anterior cruciate ligament; MCL—medial collateral ligament; LCL—lateral collateral ligament; *—extraarticular; [+]—intraarticular.

Table 6.11

Table 6.11
Normative Values of Tibial Internal and External Rotation Peak Torque (in ft-lb)

Study and population	Sex	Age	Dominant side tibial internal rotation	Nondominant side tibial internal rotation	Dominant side tibial external rotation	Nondominant side tibial external rotation
Osternig et al. (1980)						
Nondisabled	M	18-35				
30 deg/s*			89.7	102.7	101.3	111.4
30 deg/s+			78.1	77.4	83.2	81.0
Hester & Falkel (1984)						
Nondisabled	M	18-35				
30 deg/s			28.0	24.7	28.2	25.6
60 deg/s			25.4	22.8	25.6	24.1
120 deg/s			20.0	18.5	20.1	19.2
180 deg/s			16.2	15.1	16.9	15.5

Note. *—knee at 90 deg of flexion; +—knee at 45 deg of flexion.

Table 6.12

Table 6.12
Normative Values of Ankle Plantar Flexion and Dorsiflexion Peak Torque (in ft-lb)

Study and population	Sex	Age	Dominant side plantar flexion	Nondominant side plantar flexion	Dominant side dorsiflexion	Nondominant side dorsiflexion
			15 deg/s			
Oberg et al. (1987) Nondisabled (Dom = right side; NDom = left side)	M	34	108.4	147.5	27.3	40.0
			30 deg/s			
Falkel (1978) Nondisabled	M	6-8	6.6			
	F	6-8	11.4			
	M	14-16	26.5			
	F	14-16	25.1			
	M	23-28	52.4			
	F	23-28	33.3			
Fugl-Meyer et al. (1979) Nondisabled	M	30	90.7	97.4		
Fugl-Meyer (1981) Athletes	M	24	135.7		25.8	
Sedentary controls	M	25	92.9		24.3	
Poulmedis (1985) Elite soccer players	M	28	88.5		23.6	
Berg et al. (1985) College basketball players	F	20	58.3	59.9	22.8	22.4
Oberg et al. (1987) Nondisabled (Dom = right side; NDom = left side)	M	34	102.5	123.9	25.8	29.5
Seymour & Bacharach (1990) Trained subjects	F	25	55.2 42.4*			
Untrained subjects	F	25	45.5 26.4*			
Alexander (1990) Elite sprinters (Dom = average of left and right limb scores)	M	22	76.0		25.1	
		(E)	80.4		32.5	
	F	20	62.7		18.4	
		(E)	69.3		23.6	

Table 6.12 *(continued)*

Study and population	Sex	Age	Dominant side plantar flexion	Nondominant side plantar flexion	Dominant side dorsiflexion	Nondominant side dorsiflexion
60 deg/s						
Fugl-Meyer et al. (1979)						
Nondisabled	M	30	67.1	74.5		
Fugl-Meyer (1981)						
Athletes	M	24	106.9		19.9	
Sedentary controls	M	25	70.8		18.4	
Berg et al. (1985)						
College basketball players	F	20	45.3	46.9	19.8	19.4
Oberg et al. (1987)						
Nondisabled (Dom = right side; NDom = left side)	M	34	75.2	94.4	24.3	26.6
90 deg/s						
Poulmedis (1985)						
Elite soccer players	M	28	46.5		11.8	
Berg et al. (1985)						
College basketball players	F	20	36.2	36.7	17.8	17.1
120 deg/s						
Fugl-Meyer et al. (1979)						
Nondisabled	M	30	42.2	46.7		
Fugl-Meyer (1981)						
Athletes	M	24	70.1		14.8	
Sedentary controls	M	25	44.3		12.5	
Berg et al. (1985)						
College basketball players	F	20	25.9	26.2	14.0	14.1
Oberg et al. (1987)						
Nondisabled (Dom = right side; NDom = left side)	M	34	53.8	68.6	20.7	24.3
150 deg/s						
Berg et al. (1985)						
College basketball players	F	20	17.9	18.1	10.5	10.5

(continued)

Table 6.12 *(continued)*

Study and population	Sex	Age	Dominant side plantar flexion	Nondominant side plantar flexion	Dominant side dorsiflexion	Nondominant side dorsiflexion
Alexander (1990)						
Elite sprinters (Dom =	M	22	85.6		24.3	
average of left and right		(E)	93.7		34.7	
limb scores)	F	20	69.3		19.2	
		(E)	76.0		25.8	
180 deg/s						
Fugl-Meyer et al. (1979)						
Nondisabled	M	30	26.6	31.0		
Fugl-Meyer (1981)						
Athletes	M	24	46.5		12.5	
Sedentary controls	M	25	30.2		8.9	
Poulmedis (1985)						
Elite soccer players	M	28	14.0		3.7	
Oberg et al. (1987)						
Nondisabled (Dom = right side; NDom = left side)	M	34	39.1	50.2	18.4	19.2
Seymour & Bacharach (1990)						
Trained subjects	F	25	16.7 13.7*			
Untrained subjects	F	25	11.5 8.8*			
240 deg/s						
Oberg et al. (1987)						
Nondisabled (Dom = right side; NDom = left side)	M	34	28.0	37.6	15.5	14.8

Note. Plantar flexion and dorsiflexion tested with knee in extended position unless noted otherwise; Dom—dominant; NDom—nondominant; *—knee at 90 deg of flexion; E—eccentric.

Table 6.13
Normative Values of Ankle Dorsiflexion/Plantar Flexion Reciprocal Muscle Group Ratios (Percent)

Study and population	Sex	Age	Dominant dorsiflexion/plantar flexion ratio	Nondominant dorsiflexion/plantar flexion ratio
30 deg/s				
Berg et al. (1985)				
College basketball players	F	20	.39	.37
Poulmedis (1985)				
Elite soccer players	M	28	.28	
Tabin et al. (1985)				
Prepubescent (PreP) and post-	F	PreP	.30	
pubescent (PstP) athletes	M	PreP	.32	
	F	PstP	.28	
	M	PstP	.32	
Alexander (1990)				
Elite sprinters (Dom = average of	M	22	.33	
left and right limb scores)		(E)	.41	
	F	20	.31	
		(E)	.35	
60 deg/s				
Berg et al. (1985)				
College basketball players	F	20	.44	.43
90 deg/s				
Berg et al. (1985)				
College basketball players	F	20	.49	.46
120 deg/s				
Berg et al. (1985)				
College basketball players	F	20	.54	.54
150 deg/s				
Berg et al. (1985)				
College basketball players	F	20	.60	.59
Alexander (1990)				
Elite sprinters (Dom = average of	M	22	.28	
left and right limb scores)		(E)	.37	
	F	20	.28	
		(E)	.33	

Note. Dom—dominant; E—eccentric.

Table 6.14
Normative Values of Ankle Inversion and Eversion Peak Torque (in ft-lb)

Study and population	Sex	Age	Dominant inversion	Nondominant inversion	Dominant eversion	Nondominant eversion
30 deg/s						
Wong et al. (1984)						
Nondisabled	M	29	23.9	24.1	30.0	19.9
	F	28	17.6	17.5	14.7	12.4
Leslie et al. (1990)						
Nondisabled (* = 0 deg	F	27	19.4*	19.0*	15.3*	15.6*
plantar flexion; + = 20 deg			18.7+	20.0+	16.7+	14.8+
plantar flexion)						
60 deg/s						
Wong et al. (1984)						
Nondisabled	M	29	20.0	21.7	18.1	17.7
	F	28	14.7	15.6	12.1	11.2
120 deg/s						
Wong et al. (1984)						
Nondisabled	M	29	16.7	17.5	14.5	14.1
	F	28	11.9	12.6	10.1	9.6
Leslie et al. (1990)						
Nondisabled (* = 0 deg	F	27	14.2*	12.8*	8.8*	8.4*
plantar flexion; + = 20 deg			12.8+	13.6+	9.2+	8.5+
plantar flexion)						
160 deg/s						
Cawthorn et al. (1991)						
Nondisabled (* = 10 deg	F and M	21-37	17.7*		15.0*	
plantar flexion; ** = 10			14.5**		12.6**	
deg dorsiflexion; + = neutral)			16.2+		14.0+	

Table 6.15
Normative Values of Ankle Eversion/Inversion Reciprocal Muscle Group Ratios (Percent)

Study and population	Sex	Age	Dominant eversion/inversion ratio	Nondominant eversion/inversion ratio
30 deg/s				
Wong et al. (1984)				
Nondisabled	M	29	.87	
	F	28	.81	
Leslie et al. (1990)				
Nondisabled (* = 0 deg plantar	F	27	.79*	.82*
flexion; + = 20 deg plantar flexion)			.89+	.74+
60 deg/s				
Wong et al. (1984)				
Nondisabled	M	29	.90	
	F	28	.80	
120 deg/s				
Wong et al. (1984)				
Nondisabled	M	29	.86	
	F	28	.83	
Leslie et al. (1990)				
Nondisabled (* = 0 deg plantar	F	27	.62*	.65*
flexion; + = 20 deg plantar			.73+	.62+
flexion)				

Table 6.16
Test-Retest Reliability Coefficients for Lower Extremity Isokinetic Assessment of Peak Torque

Study and population	Velocity (deg/s)	Test position	Dominant correlation coefficient	Nondominant correlation coefficient
Hip flexion				
Burnett et al. (1990)				
6-10 year old boys; Kin-Com;	30 (C)	supine	.63	
(ICC)	90 (C)	supine	.75	
Hip extension				
Burnett et al. (1990)				
6-10 year old boys; Kin-Com;	30 (C)	supine	.68	
(ICC)	90 (C)	supine	.84	
Hip abduction				
Burnett et al. (1990)				
6-10 year old boys; Kin-Com;	30 (C)	laying on side	.59	
(ICC)	90 (C)	laying on side	.59	
Hip adduction				
Burnett et al. (1990)				
6-10 year old boys; Kin-Com;	30 (C)	laying on side	.55	
(ICC)	90 (C)	laying on side	.49	
Knee extension				
Johnson & Siegel (1978)				
Nondisabled; women; Cybex;	180 (C)	seated	.93-.99	
(ICC)				
Perrin (1986)				
Nondisabled; men; Cybex	60 (C)	seated	.85	.84
(GC); (r)	180 (C)	seated	.87	.93
Burdett & VanSwearingen (1987)				
Nondisabled; Cybex (GC); (ICC)	180 (C)	seated	.93	
	240 (C)	seated	.95	
Harding et al. (1988)				
Nondisabled; women; Kin-Com	60 (C)	seated	.95	
(GC); (ICC)				

Table **6.16** (*continued*)

Study and population	Velocity (deg/s)	Test position	Dominant correlation coefficient	Nondominant correlation coefficient
Knee extension				
Tredinnick & Duncan (1988)				
Nondisabled; men; Kin-Com; (ICC)	60 (C)	supine	.89	
	60 (E)	supine	.47	
	120 (C)	supine	.97	
	120 (E)	supine	.84	
	180 (C)	supine	.75	
	180 (E)	supine	.79	
Klopfer & Greij (1988)				
Nondisabled; men and women;	300 (C)	seated	.97	
Biodex (GC); (r)	450 (C)	seated	.96	
Bohannon & Smith (1989)				
Nondisabled; men and women;	60 (C)	seated	.96*	
Cybex (* = 30 deg and + = 45 deg	60 (C)	seated	.97+	
angle-specific torque) (GC); (ICC)				
Montgomery et al. (1989)				
Nondisabled; men and women;	90 (C)	seated	.92	
Biodex (GC); (ICC)	150 (C)	seated	.91	
	210 (C)	seated	.86	
	270 (C)	seated	.83	
	330 (C)	seated	.87	
Thigpen et al. (1990)				
Nondisabled; men and women;	60 (C)	seated	.96*	
Cybex (* = values from data reduc-	60 (C)	seated	.97+	
tion computer; + = values from	240 (C)	seated	.99*	
strip chart recorder); (ICC)	240 (C)	seated	.98+	
Feiring et al. (1990)				
Nondisabled; women and men;	60 (C)	seated	.95	
Biodex (GC); (ICC)	180 (C)	seated	.96	
	240 (C)	seated	.95	
	300 (C)	seated	.97	
Kramer (1990)				
Nondisabled; women; Kin-Com	45 (C)	seated	.88	
(GC); (ICC)	45 (E)	seated	.86	
	90 (C)	seated	.86	
	90 (E)	seated	.88	

(continued)

Table 6.16 *(continued)*

Study and population	Velocity (deg/s)	Test position	Dominant correlation coefficient	Nondominant correlation coefficient
Kramer (1990)				
Nondisabled; men; Kin-Com (GC); (ICC) 45 (E) seated .87	45 (C) seated .91			
	90 (C)	seated	.88	
	90 (E)	seated	.86	
Molczyk et al. (1991)				
Nondisabled; women; Cybex	60 (C)	seated	.95	.98
(values are the highest obtained	180 (C)	seated	.92	.96
from two testers) (GC); (ICC)	300 (C)	seated	.95	.95
Gross et al. (1991)				
Nondisabled; men and women;	60 (C)	seated	.97*	
* = Biodex; + = Cybex; (ICC)	60 (C)	seated	.89+	
	180 (C)	seated	.97*	
	180 (C)	seated	.87+	
Durand et al. (1991)				
Patients (men) with partial medial	30 (C)	seated	.86	
meniscal tear; DCC = injured	180 (C)	seated	.67	
extremity; Kin-Com (GC); (ICC)				
Nondisabled (men) controls;	30 (C)	seated	.87	
Kin-Com (GC); (ICC)	180 (C)	seated	.95	
Wilhite et al. (1992)				
Nondisabled; women and men;	60 (C)	seated	.76	
Kin-Com; (ICC)	60 (E)	seated	.94	
	120 (C)	seated	.85	
	120 (E)	seated	.85	
	180 (C)	seated	.80	
	180 (E)	seated	.94	
Kues et al. (1992)				
Nondisabled; women;	30 (C)	supine	.94	
Kin-Com (GC); (ICC)	30 (E)	supine	.87	
	90 (C)	supine	.94	
	90 (E)	supine	.95	
	120 (C)	supine	.98	
	120 (E)	supine	.96	
	180 (C)	supine	.98	
	180 (E)	supine	.96	

Table 6.16 *(continued)*

Study and population	Velocity (deg/s)	Test position	Dominant correlation coefficient	Nondominant correlation coefficient
		Knee flexion		
Perrin (1986)				
Nondisabled; men; Cybex	60 (C)	seated	.92	.83
(GC); (r)	180 (C)	seated	.89	.88
Burdett & VanSwearingen (1987)				
Nondisabled; Cybex (GC); (ICC)	180 (C)	seated	.81	
	240 (C)	seated	.66	
Harding et al. (1988)				
Nondisabled women; Kin-Com	60 (C)	seated	.95	
(GC); (ICC)				
Klopfer & Greij (1988)				
Nondisabled; men and women;	300 (C)	seated	.96	
Biodex (GC); (r)	450 (C)	seated	.95	
Montgomery et al. (1989)				
Nondisabled; men and women;	90 (C)	seated	.88	
Biodex (GC); (ICC)	150 (C)	seated	.86	
	210 (C)	seated	.86	
	270 (C)	seated	.75	
	330 (C)	seated	.58	
Thigpen et al. (1990)				
Nondisabled; men and women;	60 (C)	seated	.95*	
Cybex (* = values from data reduc-	60 (C)	seated	.98[+]	
tion computer; [+] = values from	240 (C)	seated	.97*	
strip chart recorder); (ICC)	240 (C)	seated	.97[+]	
Feiring et al. (1990)				
Nondisabled; women and men;	60 (C)	seated	.98	
Biodex (GC); (ICC)	180 (C)	seated	.93	
	240 (C)	seated	.93	
	300 (C)	seated	.82	
Kramer (1990)				
Nondisabled; women; Kin-Com	45 (C)	seated	.83	
(GC); (ICC)	45 (E)	seated	.82	
	90 (C)	seated	.81	
	90 (E)	seated	.79	
Nondisabled; men; Kin-Com	45 (C)	seated	.87	
(GC); (ICC)	45 (E)	seated	.80	
	90 (C)	seated	.87	
	90 (E)	seated	.86	

(continued)

Table 6.16 *(continued)*

Study and population	Velocity (deg/s)	Test position	Dominant correlation coefficient	Nondominant correlation coefficient
Molczyk et al. (1991)				
Nondisabled; women; Cybex	60 (C)	seated	.95	.95
(values are the highest obtained	180 (C)	seated	.89	.92
from two testers) (GC); (ICC)	300 (C)	seated	.89	.90
Gross et al. (1991)				
Nondisabled; men and women;	60 (C)	seated	.95*	
* = Biodex; + = Cybex; (ICC)	60 (C)	seated	.86+	
	180 (C)	seated	.77*	
	180 (C)	seated	.86+	
Durand et al. (1991)				
Patients (men) with partial	30 (C)	seated	.87	
medial meniscal tear; DCC =	180 (C)	seated	.92	
injured extremity; Kin-Com				
(GC); (ICC)				
Nondisabled (men) controls;	30 (C)	seated	.64	
Kin-Com (GC); (ICC)	180 (C)	seated	.79	

Ankle plantar flexion

Karnofel et al. (1989)				
Nondisabled; men and women;	60 (C)	45 deg knee flexion	.91	
Cybex; (r)	120 (C)	45 deg knee flexion	.94	
Wennerberg (1991)				
Athletes; men; Biodex; (r)	30 (C)	45 deg knee flexion	.68	
	120 (C)	45 deg knee flexion	.78	

Ankle dorsiflexion

Karnofel et al. (1989)				
Nondisabled; men and women;	60 (C)	45 deg knee flexion	.86	
Cybex; (r)	120 (C)	45 deg knee flexion	.89	
Wennerberg (1991)				
Athletes; men; Biodex; (r)	30 (C)	45 deg knee flexion	.79	
	120 (C)	45 deg knee flexion	.67	

Ankle inversion

Karnofel et al. (1989)				
Nondisabled; men and women;	60 (C)	15 deg knee flexion	.91	
Cybex; (r)	120 (C)	15 deg knee flexion	.91	

Table 6.16 *(continued)*

Study and population	Velocity (deg/s)	Test position	Dominant correlation coefficient	Nondominant correlation coefficient
Cawthorn et al. (1991)				
Nondisabled; men and women;	160 (C)	10 deg ankle PF	.94	
Merac; (r)		10 deg ankle DF	.91	
		ankle neutral	.92	
Ankle eversion				
Karnofel et al. (1989)				
Nondisabled; men and women;	60 (C)	15 deg knee flexion	.78	
Cybex; (r)	120 (C)	15 deg knee flexion	.89	
Cawthorn et al. (1991)				
Nondisabled; men and women;	160 (C)	10 deg ankle PF	.90	
Merac; (r)		10 deg ankle DF	.89	
		ankle neutral	.87	

Note. C—concentric; E—eccentric; ICC—intraclass correlation coefficient; GC—gravity correction procedure used; r—Pearson product-moment correlation coefficient; PF—plantar flexion; DF—dorsiflexion; DCC—dominant correlation coefficient.

Chapter 7

Isokinetic Assessment and Exercise of the Trunk

Both clinicians and researchers can now assess isokinetic muscle performance of the trunk. In this chapter I discuss the concepts important for safe, accurate assessment of these muscles. While less expansive than those for either the upper or lower extremity, the tables at the end of the chapter present the normative and reliability data that currently exist for the trunk.

THE TRUNK

The joints of the trunk consist of the articulation of each vertebra with its adjacent superior and inferior vertebrae. The movement at each articulation of the cervical, thoracic, and lumbar vertebrae is somewhat limited, yet movement across all of these vertebrae permits motion through each of the cardinal planes. The sacral and coccygeal vertebrae are fused and thus do not permit movement.

Assessment of trunk strength is important among athletes but may be more valuable for industrial workers, given their extremely high incidence of back pain. Most individuals have been found to have 48% to 82% greater trunk flexion and extension strength than patients with chronic dysfunction of the lower back (Smidt et al., 1983). This finding underscores the importance of screening patients for strength of the trunk musculature and implementing appropriate exercise programs for those with deficits. Isokinetic assessment already plays a particularly important role in industrial work-hardening programs and could greatly improve the process of prescreening applicants for rigorous manual labor. Isokinetic exercise of the trunk might play a valuable role in the application of mechanical stresses to vertebrae

175

to improve bone health and prevent or delay development of osteoporosis. Indeed, more research is needed to establish normative data and to explore the value of isokinetic assessment and exercise of the trunk flexor and extensor musculature.

Because of the multiplicity of joints in the spine, alignment of joints with dynamometer axes of rotation is more complex than in most joints of the extremities. Depending on preference, the point of alignment ranges from L1-L2 to the greater trochanter of the femur (Grabiner, Jeziorowski, & Divekar, 1990). The L5-S1 level is most frequently used for alignment of trunk and dynamometer axes of rotation; locate it by palpating the posterior superior iliac supine and then moving 1 in. superiorly (Davies & Gould, 1982).

Trunk Flexion and Extension

Flexion and extension of the trunk occur through the sagittal plane (Figure 7.1, a and b). The primary flexors of the trunk include the abdominal group— the rectus abdominis, external oblique, and internal oblique muscles. Contribution from muscles acting on the hip may also influence trunk flexor strength. Indeed, if assessed from the standing position, the iliopsoas can approximately double the strength of the trunk flexors (Langrana & Lee,

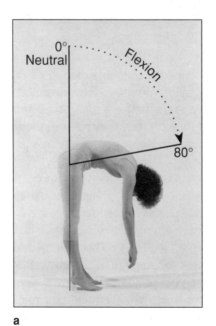
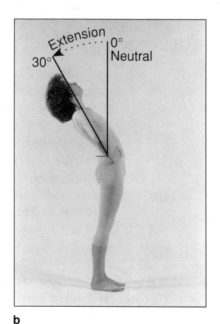

Figure 7.1 Trunk flexion (a) and extension (b) range of motion.

1984). Extension of the trunk is accomplished by contraction of a number of paired muscles known as the erector spinae—the iliocostalis thoracis, iliocostalis lumborum, longissimus thoracis, and spinalis thoracis muscles.

Isokinetic strength of the lumbar flexors and extensors has been assessed from standing (Figure 7.2), seated (Figure 7.3), prone, supine, and side-lying positions. Muscles controlling the trunk relative to the lower extremity (i.e., muscles acting on the hip) can confound the assessment of muscles acting on the trunk (Thorstensson & Nilsson, 1982), so your goal in positioning is to minimize contribution from muscles acting on the hip and to attain maximal stabilization of the pelvic girdle. The seated position seems to best foster these goals (Langrana & Lee, 1984).

Table 7.1 presents normative data for the trunk flexor and extensor muscles when assessed from a variety of test positions in nondisabled and athletic men and women and in healthy and chronic back-pain patients. Interpretation of "normal" values for these muscle groups is somewhat more complex than for muscles of the extremities because comparison with a contralateral side is impossible. In general, the effects of increases in velocity and changes in the length-tension relationship are similar to the muscles of the extremities (Thorstensson & Nilsson, 1982). For example, concentric peak torque values tend to decrease with increases in test velocity. Very few reports of eccentric strength of the trunk flexor and extensor muscles can be found in the scientific literature. More research is needed to determine if the eccentric force-velocity relationship of the trunk muscles responds in a fashion similar to muscle groups of the extremities. Test position also influences normative strength values of the trunk. I advise the reader to note the test position, the potential effects of gravity in the various test positions, and the population from which the normative values were obtained.

Trunk strength is frequently expressed as a percentage of total body weight. In general, men tend to produce more torque relative to body weight than women for the trunk flexors and extensors. For both men and women, this percentage decreases with increases in test velocity. In general, men tend to exceed 100% of total body weight with the trunk extensor muscle group at slow test velocities, and athletic women have also exceeded 100%. The strength of the trunk flexor muscles relative to body weight is related to test position. When assessed from a standing position, peak torque of the flexors usually exceeds 80% of total body weight in both men and women, but this percentage is substantially reduced if assessment is from a seated position. Table 7.2 presents strength of the trunk flexor and extensor muscles relative to total body weight.

Table 7.3 presents normative reciprocal muscle group ratios for the trunk musculature. The trunk extensors tend to produce more torque than the

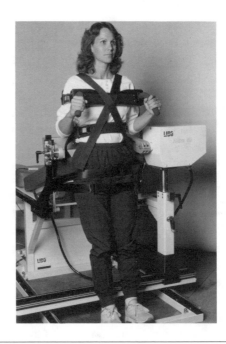

Figure 7.2 Test and exercise position for the trunk flexor and extensor muscles while standing.

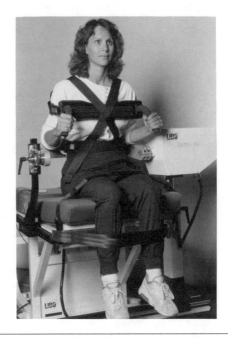

Figure 7.3 Test and exercise position for the trunk flexor and extensor muscles while seated.

flexors, yet trunk flexion torque appears to approach and then exceed extension torque as test velocity increases (Thompson, Gould, Davies, Ross, & Price, 1985). This phenomenon may be related to the absence of a gravity correction procedure in virtually all reports of trunk flexion and extension strength in the literature. For example, a similar phenomenon is seen with the knee flexor/extensor reciprocal muscle group ratio in the absence of a gravity correction procedure. The hamstring muscle group's increase in strength relative to the quadriceps is reduced with increases in test velocity when a gravity correction procedure is employed. In any event, I recommend assessment and exercise of the trunk at slower velocities because the substantial mass of the trunk makes acceleration to higher velocities difficult. Interpretation of the values from Table 7.3 is somewhat complicated because of the variations in method of determining reciprocal muscle group ratio. For example, some reports calculate a trunk flexor/extensor ratio; others report an extensor/flexor ratio. Some simply state the relationship of extension to flexion (i.e., an extensor:flexor ratio). Interpretation of the trunk reciprocal muscle group ratio is simplified when determined simply by dividing the muscle group that is usually weakest by the muscle group that is usually strongest (i.e., a trunk flexor/extensor ratio). Moreover, this method is consistent with the technique most often used to express reciprocal muscle group ratios of the upper and lower extremities.

The effect of gravity on trunk assessment can be particularly significant because the trunk constitutes more than 50% of the total mass of the body (Thorstensson & Nilsson, 1982). Gravity correction is especially important if the trunk is raised from a horizontal position (Hasue, Fujiwara, & Kikuchi, 1980). The effect of gravity would be essentially eliminated if trunk flexion and extension were assessed in the horizontal plane (Andersson, Sward, & Thorstensson, 1988; Thorstensson & Nilsson, 1982), but most contemporary isokinetic dynamometry cannot assess from this position. Assessment of flexion and extension from the seated position permits motion that is nearly equal on either side of the vertical plane, so gravity correction may not be essential when assessing from this position (Smidt et al., 1983). Further research is needed to determine the effects of gravity in assessment of trunk muscle strength from a variety of test positions.

Trunk Rotation

Rotation of the trunk occurs through the transverse plane of the body (Figure 7.4) and is produced primarily by the internal and external oblique abdominal muscles. The internal oblique produces rotation to the same side, and the external oblique to the opposite side (Rasch &

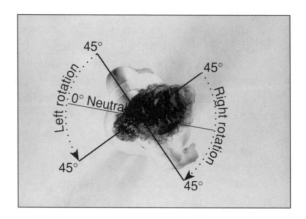

Figure 7.4   Trunk rotation range of motion.

Burke, 1978). Thus, the right internal oblique and the left external oblique rotate to the right, and the left internal oblique and the right external oblique rotate to the left. Although both contralateral and ipsilateral obliques contract during rotation, electromyographic analysis indicates the activity of the contralateral obliques is greater than the ipsilateral obliques (Mayer et al., 1985).

Very little normative data are available for the trunk rotator muscle groups, probably because of the limited number of isokinetic dynamometers that can assess this motion. Table 7.4 presents values of left and right rotation at four test velocities for an athletic population. Table 7.5 presents left and right rotation reciprocal muscle group ratios for a population of nondisabled subjects at four test velocities. In general, we see little difference between the left and right rotator muscle groups. Further research is needed to describe the strength of these muscle groups in a variety of athletic and nonathletic (nondisabled) populations.

Trunk Lateral Flexion

Lateral flexion of the trunk to the right and left sides occurs in the frontal plane (Figure 7.5). The paraspinal and abdominal muscles all assist in producing lateral flexion to the same side, although the quadratus lumborum muscle is the only "true" lateral flexor of the spine. As with the trunk rotator muscles, little normative data is available for lateral flexion of the trunk. Table 7.6 presents normative values for left and right lateral trunk flexion for both nondisabled and low-back-pain subjects. Little difference exists between left and right lateral flexion in normal subjects, although some athletes tend to have higher lateral flexion values on the nondominant side (Andersson et al., 1988).

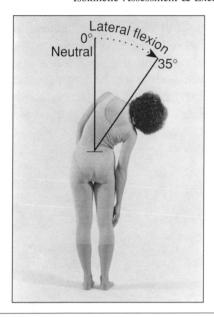

Figure 7.5   Trunk lateral flexion range of motion.

RELIABILITY OF TRUNK ASSESSMENT

Although most normative data for the trunk musculature have been obtained with the subjects standing, supine, prone, or laying on their sides, published data of reliability of assessment are reported only for the seated test position. Table 7.7 presents reliability of assessing the trunk flexor and extensor musculature in healthy and in low-back-pain subjects. For assessment of trunk flexion, the reliability coefficients tend to be higher in healthy subjects than in back-pain patients. Interestingly, test velocity appears to have an inverse effect on these two populations. Reliability tends to decrease with increases in test velocity in the healthy subjects, whereas the opposite seems to occur in the low-back-pain patients. This trend might be related to several factors. Maximal extension of the spine at slow testing velocities can be extremely painful in individuals experiencing facet joint osteoarthritis secondary to loss of disk height and integrity with aging. If a reduction in compressive forces at the intervertebral joints is associated with increases in test velocity, exercise and assessment might be more comfortable for these patients. During assessment of trunk flexion, patients with diskogenic etiology of low back pain might be more comfortable with the less forceful muscular contraction associated with more rapid movement. Additional research is needed to explore this potential phenomenon as well as the role of range of motion through which isokinetic assessment occurs in both healthy and low-back-pain subjects. Reliability of trunk extensor assessment appears to be quite good and consistent regardless of test velocity in normal subjects, although a trend seems to exist toward better reliability at higher test velocities in low back pain subjects. Reliability of eccentric trunk flexion and extension has not been established. Moreover, virtually no reports of reliability of either concentric or eccentric trunk rotation or lateral flexion exist.

Table 7.1
Normative Values of Trunk Flexion and Extension Peak Torque (in ft-lb)

Study and population	Sex	Age	Flexion	Extension
6 deg/s				
Hasue et al. (1980)				
Nondisabled (extension assessed prone)	M	10-19		140.9
		20-29		149.0
		30-39		141.5
		40-49		116.8
		50-59		100.8
	F	10-19		87.9
		20-29		99.0
		30-39		97.1
		40-49		87.9
		50-59		54.6
12 deg/s				
Hasue et al. (1980)				
Nondisabled (flexion assessed supine)	M	10-19	119.8	
		20-29	130.3	
		30-39	116.7	
		40-49	87.1	
		50-59	79.4	
	F	10-19	72.4	
		20-29	68.1	
		30-39	65.5	
		40-49	57.0	
		50-59	30.3	
15 deg/s				
Thorstensson & Nilsson (1982)				
Nondisabled (assessed laying on side)	M	23	67.1	184.4
Thorstensson & Arvidson (1982)				
Low-back-pain patients* and non-disabled (assessed laying on side)	M*	19-20	50.2	154.9
	M	19-21	60.5	162.3
Tis et al. (1991)				
Runners (assessed seated; values expressed as average force in newtons)	F	30	196.7	391.4
		(E)	212.2	553.0

(continued)

Table 7.1 *(continued)*

Study and population	Sex	Age	Flexion	Extension
30 deg/s				
Thorstensson & Nilsson (1982)				
Nondisabled (assessed laying on side)	M	23	63.4	178.5
Thorstensson & Arvidson (1982)				
Low-back-pain patients* and non-	M*	19-20	46.5	144.6
disabled (assessed laying on side)	M	19-21	56.8	157.8
Davies & Gould (1982)				
Athletes (assessed standing)	M	21	184.9	229.4
	F	20	120.4	184.9
Langrana & Lee (1984)				
Nondisabled (assessed seated)	M	18-40	101.0	156.4
	F	20-45	44.3	70.1
Langrana et al. (1984)				
Nondisabled (assessed seated)	M	18-40	101.0	156.4
Nondisabled (assessed seated)	F	20-45	44.3	72.3
Patients with back disorders (assessed seated)	M and F	24-35	42.0	52.4
Thompson et al. (1985)				
Nondisabled (assessed standing)	M	43	180.2	197.3
	F	38	111.2	118.7
60 deg/s				
Davies & Gould (1982)				
Athletes (assessed standing)	M	21	181.6	199.5
	F	20	118.3	133.8
Thompson et al. (1985)				
Nondisabled (assessed standing)	M	43	183.6	191.5
	F	38	109.2	110.0
90 deg/s				
Davies & Gould (1982)				
Athletes (assessed standing)	M	21	174.0	175.6
	F	20	114.9	116.8
Thompson et al. (1985)				
Nondisabled (assessed standing)	M	43	186.6	183.3
	F	38	106.9	104.4

Table 7.1 *(continued)*

Study and population	Sex	Age	Flexion	Extension
		120 deg/s		
Davies & Gould (1982)				
Athletes (assessed standing)	M	21	161.4	109.7
	F	20	109.7	99.7
Thompson et al. (1985)				
Nondisabled (assessed standing)	M	43	187.1	179.0
	F	38	105.6	103.2

Note. E—eccentric.

Table 7.2
Normative Values of Trunk Flexion and Extension Expressed as a Percentage of Body Weight

Study and population	Sex	Age	Flexion	Extension
15 deg/s				
Andersson et al. (1988)				
Soccer players	M	22	1.52	3.63
Wrestlers	M	22	1.79	3.75
Gymnasts	M	20	1.98	3.92
	F	18	1.50	2.85
Tennis players	M	19	1.84	3.41
Nondisabled	M	20	1.30	3.40
(All subjects assessed laying on side; values expressed as Nm/kg body weight)				
30 deg/s				
Davies & Gould (1982)				
Athletes (assessed standing)	M	21	98.0	122.0
	F	20	90.0	109.0
Thompson et al. (1985)				
Nondisabled (assessed standing)	M	43	96.0	106.9
	F	38	84.2	89.8
60 deg/s				
Davies & Gould (1982)				
Athletes (assessed standing)	M	21	96.0	108.0
	F	20	89.0	96.0
Thompson et al. (1985)				
Nondisabled (assessed standing)	M	43	97.2	103.3
	F	38	82.0	83.0
Grabiner et al. (1990)				
Nondisabled (assessed seated)	F	26	40.8	91.7
90 deg/s				
Davies & Gould (1982)				
Athletes (assessed standing)	M	21	93.0	93.0
	F	20	86.0	84.0
Thompson et al. (1985)				
Nondisabled (assessed standing)	M	43	98.8	98.6
	F	38	80.0	78.9

Table 7.2 *(continued)*

Study and population	Sex	Age	Flexion	Extension
120 deg/s				
Davies & Gould (1982)				
Athletes (assessed standing)	M	21	85.0	77.0
	F	20	82.0	71.0
Thompson et al. (1985)				
Nondisabled (assessed standing)	M	43	98.9	96.4
	F	38	79.1	77.9
Grabiner et al. (1990)				
Nondisabled (assessed seated)	F	26	39.4	81.7
180 deg/s				
Grabiner et al. (1990)				
Nondisabled (assessed seated)	F	26	43.4	65.4

Table 7.3
Normative Values of Trunk Flexor and Extensor Reciprocal Muscle Group Ratios (Percent)

Study and population	Sex	Age	Ratio
15 deg/s			
Thorstensson & Nilsson (1982)			
Nondisabled (assessed laying on side; values expressed as extension/flexion ratio)	M	23	2.85
Tis et al. (1991)			
Runners (assessed seated; values expressed as flexion/extension ratio)	F	30 (E)	.52 .39
30 deg/s			
Thorstensson & Nilsson (1982)			
Nondisabled (assessed laying on side; values expressed as extension/flexion ratio)	M	23	2.93
Davies & Gould (1982)			
Athletes (assessed standing; values expressed as flexion/extension ratio)	M F	21 20	.80 .80
Thompson et al. (1985)			
Nondisabled (assessed standing; values expressed as flexion/extension ratio)	M F	43 38	.93 .97
Smith et al. (1985)			
Nondisabled (assessed standing; values expressed as extension to flexion)	M F M F	18-29 18-29 30-44 30-44	1.4:1 1.4:1 1.3:1 1.5:1
60 deg/s			
Davies & Gould (1982)			
Athletes (assessed standing; values expressed as flexion/extension ratio)	M F	21 20	.91 .88
Thompson et al. (1985)			
Nondisabled (assessed standing; values expressed as flexion/extension ratio)	M F	43 38	.97 1.02
Smith et al. (1985)			
Nondisabled (assessed standing; values expressed as extension to flexion)	M F M F	18-29 18-29 30-44 30-44	1.3:1 1.4:1 1.2:1 1.5:1

Table 7.3 *(continued)*

Study and population	Sex	Age	Ratio
90 deg/s			
Davies & Gould (1982)			
Athletes (assessed standing; values	M	21	.99
expressed as flexion/extension ratio)	F	20	.98
Thompson et al. (1985)			
Nondisabled (assessed standing; values	M	43	1.02
expressed as flexion/extension ratio)	F	38	1.06
Smith et al. (1985)			
Nondisabled (assessed standing; values	M	18-29	1.3:1
expressed as extension to flexion)	F	18-29	1.3:1
	M	30-44	1.2:1
	F	30-44	1.3:1
120 deg/s			
Davies & Gould (1982)			
Athletes (assessed standing; values	M	21	1.10
expressed as flexion/extension ratio)	F	20	1.10
Thompson et al. (1985)			
Nondisabled (assessed standing; values	M	43	1.05
expressed as flexion/extension ratio)	F	38	1.05
Smith et al. (1985)			
Nondisabled (assessed standing; values	M	18-29	1.3:1
expressed as extension to flexion)	F	18-29	1.3:1
	M	30-44	1.1:1
	F	30-44	1.2:1

Note. E—eccentric.

Table 7.4
Normative Values of Left and Right Trunk Rotation Peak Torque (in ft-lb)

Study and population	Sex	Age	Left rotation	Right rotation
Woodhouse et al. (1990)				
Athletes				
60 deg/s	M	26	142.2	135.4
90 deg/s	M	26	136.0	137.4
120 deg/s	M	26	130.6	136.0
150 deg/s	M	26	125.5	129.4

Table 7.5
Normative Values of Left and Right Trunk Rotation Reciprocal Muscle Group Ratios (Percent)

Study and population	Sex	Age	Ratio
Smith et al. (1985)			
Nondisabled			
30 deg/s	M	27	1.0:1
	F	27	1.0:1
60 deg/s	M	27	1.9:1
	F	27	1.0:1
120 deg/s	M	27	0.9:1
	F	27	1.0:1
180 deg/s	M	27	1.0:1
	F	27	1.0:1

Table 7.6
Normative Values of Trunk Lateral Flexion Peak Torque (in ft-lb)

Study and population	Sex	Age	Left flexion	Right flexion
15 deg/s				
Thorstensson & Nilsson (1982)				
Nondisabled (assessed supine)	M	23	133.5	134.2
Thorstensson & Arvidson (1982)				
Low-back-pain patients* and	M*	19-20	98.1	102.5
nondisabled (assessed supine)	M	19-21	121.0	117.3
30 deg/s				
Thorstensson & Nilsson (1982)				
Nondisabled (assessed supine)	M	23	127.6	118.0
Thorstensson & Arvidson (1982)				
Low-back-pain patients* and	M*	19-20	104.0	101.0
nondisabled (assessed supine)	M	19-21	114.3	104.0

Table 7.7
Reliability Coefficients for Isokinetic Assessment of Trunk Flexion and Extension Peak Torque

Study and population	Velocity (deg/s)	Test position	Coefficient
Flexion			
Smidt et al. (1983)			
Nondisabled; men and women; adapted Cybex (reliability for intraday strength trials); (ICC)	30	seated	.99
Grabiner et al. (1990)			
Nondisabled and low-back-pain patients*;	60	seated	.96
men; Biodex (reliability for test, retest	60	seated	.73*
trials); (ICC)	120	seated	.94
	120	seated	.86*
	180	seated	.81
	180	seated	.96*
Friedlander et al. (1991)			
Nondisabled; men and women;	60	seated	.95
Cybex; (r)	90	seated	.90
	120	seated	.92
Extension			
Smidt et al. (1983)			
Nondisabled; men and women; adapted Cybex (reliability for intraday strength trials); (ICC)	30	seated	.99
Grabiner et al. (1990)			
Nondisabled and low-back-pain patients*;	60	seated	.97
men; Biodex (reliability for test, retest	60	seated	.87*
trials); (ICC)	120	seated	.95
	120	seated	.97*
	180	seated	.96
	180	seated	.97*
Friedlander et al. (1991)			
Nondisabled; men and women;	60	seated	.88
Cybex; (r)	90	seated	.83
	120	seated	.88

Note. ICC—intraclass correlation coefficient; r—Pearson product-moment correlation coefficient.

References

Alderink, G.J., & Kuck, D.J. (1986). Isokinetic shoulder strength of high school and college-aged pitchers. *Journal of Orthopaedic and Sports Physical Therapy*, **7**, 163-172.

Alexander, M.J.L. (1990). Peak torque values for antagonist muscle groups and concentric and eccentric contraction types for elite sprinters. *Archives of Physical Medicine and Rehabilitation*, **71**, 334-339.

American College of Sports Medicine. (1991). *Guidelines for exercise testing and prescription.* Philadelphia: Lea & Febiger.

Anderson, M.A., Gieck, J.H., Perrin, D.H., Weltman, A., Rutt, R., & Denegar, C. (1991). The relationship among isometric, isotonic, and isokinetic concentric and eccentric quadriceps and hamstring force and three components of athletic performance. *Journal of Orthopaedic and Sports Physical Therapy*, **14**, 114-120.

Andersson, E., Sward, L., & Thorstensson, A. (1988). Trunk muscle strength in athletes. *Medicine and Science in Sports and Exercise*, **20**, 587-593.

Appen, L., & Duncan, P.W. (1986). Strength relationship of the knee musculature: Effects of gravity and sport. *Journal of Orthopaedic and Sports Physical Therapy*, **7**, 232-235.

Baltzopoulos, V., & Brodie, D.A. (1989). Isokinetic dynamometry: Applications and limitations. *Sports Medicine*, **8**, 101-116.

Baltzopoulos, V., Williams, J.G., & Brodie, D.A. (1991). Sources of error in isokinetic dynamometry: Effects of visual feedback on maximum torque measurements. *Journal of Orthopaedic and Sports Physical Therapy*, **13**, 138-141.

Barr, A.E., & Duncan, P.W. (1988). Influence of position on knee flexor peak torque. *Journal of Orthopaedic and Sports Physical Therapy*, **9**, 279-283.

Basmajian, J.V. (1979). *Muscles alive: Their functions revealed by electromyography.* Baltimore: Williams & Wilkins.

Baumgartner, T.A. (1989). Norm-referenced measurement: Reliability. In M.J. Safrit & T.M. Woods (Eds.), *Measurement concepts in physical education and exercise science* (pp. 45-60). Champaign, IL: Human Kinetics.

Bemben, M.G., Grump, K.J., & Massey, B.H. (1988). Assessment of technical accuracy of the Cybex II isokinetic dynamometer and analog recording system. *Journal of Orthopaedic and Sports Physical Therapy*, **10**, 12-17.

Bennett, J.G., & Stauber, W.T. (1986). Evaluation and treatment of anterior knee pain using eccentric exercise. *Medicine and Science in Sports and Exercise*, **18**, 526-530.

Berg, K., Blanke, D., & Miller, M. (1985). Muscular fitness profile of female college basketball players. *Journal of Orthopaedic and Sports Physical Therapy*, **7**, 59-64.

Bohannon, R.W., & Smith, M.B. (1989). Intrasession reliability of angle specific knee extension torque measurements with gravity corrections. *Journal of Orthopaedic and Sports Physical Therapy*, **11**, 155-157.

Brooke, M.H., & Kaiser, K.K. (1970). Muscle fiber types: How many and what kind? *Archives of Neurology*, **23**, 369-379.

Brown, L.P., Niehues, S.L., Harrah, A., Yavorsky, P., & Hirschman, H.P. (1988). Upper extremity range of motion and isokinetic strength of the internal and external shoulder rotators in major league baseball players. *American Journal of Sports Medicine*, **16**, 577-585.

Burdett, R.G., & VanSwearingen, J. (1987). Reliability of isokinetic muscle endurance tests. *Journal of Orthopaedic and Sports Physical Therapy*, **8**, 484-488.

Burnett, C.N., Betts, E.F., & King, W.M. (1990). Reliability of isokinetic measurements of hip muscle torque in young boys. *Physical Therapy*, **70**, 244-249.

Burnie, J. (1987). Factors affecting selected reciprocal muscle group ratios in preadolescents. *International Journal of Sports Medicine*, **8**, 40-45.

Campbell, D.E., & Glenn, W. (1979). Foot-pounds of torque of the normal knee and the rehabilitated postmeniscectomy knee. *Physical Therapy*, **59**, 418-421.

Cawthorn, M., Cummings, G., Walker, J.R., & Donatelli, R. (1991). Isokinetic measurement of foot invertor and evertor force in three positions of plantar flexion and dorsiflexion. *Journal of Orthopaedic and Sports Physical Therapy*, **14**, 75-81.

Chmelar, R.D., Shultz, B.B., Ruhling, R.O., Fitt, S.S., & Johnson, M.B. (1988). Isokinetic characteristics of the knee in female, professional and university, ballet and modern dancers. *Journal of Orthopaedic and Sports Physical Therapy*, **9**, 410-418.

Clarke, H.H. (1948). Objective strength tests of affected muscle groups involved with orthopedic disabilities. *Research Quarterly*, **19**, 118-147.

Colliander, E.B., & Tesch, P.A. (1989). Bilateral eccentric and concentric torque of quadriceps and hamstring muscles in females and males. *European Journal of Applied Physiology*, **59**, 227-232.

Connelly Maddux, R.E., Kibler, W.B., & Uhl, T. (1989). Isokinetic peak torque and work values for the shoulder. *Journal of Orthopaedic and Sports Physical Therapy*, **11**, 264-269.

Cook, E.E., Gray, V.L., Savinar-Nogue, E., & Medeiros, J. (1987). Shoulder antagonistic strength ratios: A comparison between college-level baseball pitchers and nonpitchers. *Journal of Orthopaedic and Sports Physical Therapy*, **8**, 451-461.

Costain, R., & Williams, A.K. (1984). Isokinetic quadriceps and hamstring torque levels of adolescent, female soccer players. *Journal of Orthopaedic and Sports Physical Therapy*, **5**, 196-200.

Costill, D.L., Coyle, E.F., Fink, W.F., Lesmes, G.R., & Witzmann, F.A. (1979). Adaptations in skeletal muscle following strength training. *Journal of Applied Physiology*, **46**, 96-99.

Cote, C., Simoneau, J.A., Lagasse, P., Boulay, M., Thibault, M.C., Marcotte, M., & Bouchard, C. (1988). Isokinetic strength training protocols: Do they induce skeletal muscle fiber hypertrophy? *Archives of Physical Medicine and Rehabilitation*, **69**, 281-285.

Coyle, E.F., Feiring, D.C., Rotkis, T.C., Cote, R.W., Roby, F.B., Lee, W., & Wilmore, J.H. (1981). Specificity of power improvements through slow and fast isokinetic training. *Journal of Applied Physiology*, **51**, 1437-1442.

Croce, R.V. (1986). The effects of EMG biofeedback on strength acquisition. *Biofeedback and Self-Regulation*, **11**, 299-310.

Daniels, L., & Worthingham, C. (1980). *Muscle testing: Techniques of manual examination.* Philadelphia: W.B. Saunders.

Davies, G.J., & Gould, J.A. (1982). Trunk testing using a prototype Cybex II isokinetic dynamometer stabilization system. *Journal of Orthopaedic and Sports Physical Therapy*, **3**, 164-170.

Day, R.W., Moore, R.J., & Patterson, P. (1988). Isokinetic torque production of the shoulder in a functional movement pattern. *Athletic Training*, **23**, 333-338.

Dibrezzo, R., Gench, B.E., Hinson, M.M., & King, J. (1985). Peak torque values of the knee extensor and flexor muscles of females. *Journal of Orthopaedic and Sports Physical Therapy*, **7**, 65-68.

Donatelli, R., Catlin, P.A., Backer, G.S., Drane, D.L., & Slater, S.M. (1991). Isokinetic hip abductor to adductor torque ratio in normals. *Isokinetics and Exercise Science*, **1**, 103-111.

Douris, P.C. (1991). Cardiovascular responses to velocity-specific isokinetic exercise. *Journal of Orthopaedic and Sports Physical Therapy*, **13**, 28-32.

Duncan, P.W., Chandler, J., Cavanaugh, D., Johnson, K., & Buehler, S. (1989). Mode and speed specificity of eccentric and concentric exercise. *Journal of Orthopaedic and Sports Physical Therapy*, **11**, 70-75.

Durand, A., Malouin, F., Richards, C.L., & Bravo, G. (1991). Intertrial reliability of work measurements recorded during concentric isokinetic knee extension and flexion in subjects with and without meniscal tears. *Physical Therapy*, **71**, 804-812.

Ellenbecker, T.S., Davies, G.J., & Rowinski, M.J. (1988). Concentric versus eccentric isokinetic strengthening of the rotator cuff. *American Journal of Sports Medicine*, **16**, 64-69.

Engle, B. (1983). Clinical use of an isokinetic leg press. *Journal of Orthopaedic and Sports Physical Therapy*, **4**, 148-149.

Falkel, J. (1978). Plantar flexor strength testing using the Cybex isokinetic dynamometer. *Physical Therapy*, **58**, 847-850.

Farrell, M., & Richards, J.G. (1986). Analysis of the reliability and validity of the kinetic communicator exercise device. *Medicine and Science in Sports and Exercise*, **18**, 44-49.

Feiring, D.C., Ellenbecker, T.S., & Derscheid, G.L. (1990). Test-retest reliability of the Biodex isokinetic dynamometer. *Journal of Orthopaedic and Sports Physical Therapy*, **11**, 298-300.

Figoni, S.F., Christ, C.B., & Massey, B.H. (1988). Effects of speed, hip and knee angle, and gravity on hamstring to quadriceps torque ratios. *Journal of Orthopaedic and Sports Physical Therapy*, **9**, 287-291.

Figoni, S.F., & Morris, A.F. (1984). Effects of knowledge of results on reciprocal, isokinetic strength and fatigue. *Journal of Orthopaedic and Sports Physical Therapy*, **6**, 190-197.

Fillyaw, M., Bevins, T., & Fernandez, L. (1986). Importance of correcting isokinetic peak torque for the effect of gravity when calculating knee flexor to extensor muscle ratios. *Physical Therapy*, **66**, 23-29.

Friedlander, A.L., Block, J.E., Byl, N.N., Stubbs, H.A., Sadowsky, H.S., & Genant, H.K. (1991). Isokinetic limb and trunk muscle performance testing: Short-term reliability. *Journal of Orthopaedic and Sports Physical Therapy*, **14**, 220-224.

Fugl-Meyer, A.R. (1981). Maximum isokinetic ankle plantar and dorsal flexion torques in trained subjects. *European Journal of Applied Physiology*, **47**, 393-404.

Fugl-Meyer, A.R., Sjostrom, M., & Wahlby, L. (1979). Human plantar flexion strength and structure. *Acta Physiologica Scandinavica*, **107**, 47-56.

Ghena, D.R., Kurth, A.L., Thomas, M., & Mayhew, J. (1991). Torque characteristics of the quadriceps and hamstring muscles during concentric and eccentric loading. *Journal of Orthopaedic and Sports Physical Therapy*, **14**, 149-154.

Gilliam, T.B., Villanacci, J.F., Freedson, P.S., & Sady, S.P. (1979). Isokinetic torque in boys and girls ages 7 to 13: Effect of age, height, and weight. *Research Quarterly*, **50**, 599-609.

Grabiner, M.D., Jeziorowski, J.J., & Divekar, A.D. (1990). Isokinetic measurements of trunk extension and flexion performance collected with the Biodex clinical data station. *Journal of Orthopaedic and Sports Physical Therapy*, **11**, 590-598.

Green, H.J. (1986). Muscle power: Fibre type recruitment, metabolism and fatigue. In N.L. Jones, N. McCartney, & A.J. McComas (Eds.), *Human muscle power* (pp. 65-79). Champaign, IL: Human Kinetics.

Greenfield, B.H., Donatelli, R., Wooden, M.J., & Wilkes, J. (1990). Isokinetic evaluation of shoulder rotational strength between the plane of scapula and the frontal plane. *American Journal of Sports Medicine*, **18**, 124-128.

Griffin, J.W. (1987). Differences in elbow flexion torque measured concentrically, eccentrically, and isometrically. *Physical Therapy*, **67**, 1205-1209.

Gross, M.T., Huffman, G.M., Phillips, C.N., & Wray, J.A. (1991). Intramachine and intermachine reliability of the Biodex and Cybex II for knee flexion and extension peak torque and angular work. *Journal of Orthopaedic and Sports Physical Therapy*, **13**, 329-335.

Guth, L., & Samaha, F.J. (1969). Qualitative differences between actomyosin ATPase of slow and fast mammalian muscle. *Experimental Neurology*, **25**, 139-152.

Hageman, P.A., Gillaspie, D.M., & Hill, L.D. (1988). Effects of speed and limb dominance on eccentric and concentric isokinetic testing of the knee. *Journal of Orthopaedic and Sports Physical Therapy*, **10**, 59-65.

Hageman, P.A., Mason, D.K., Rydlund, K.W., & Humpal, S.A. (1989). Effects of position and speed on eccentric and concentric isokinetic testing of the shoulder rotators. *Journal of Orthopaedic and Sports Physical Therapy*, **11**, 64-69.

Hald, R.D., & Bottjen, E.J. (1987). Effect of visual feedback on maximal and submaximal isokinetic test measurements of normal quadriceps and hamstrings. *Journal of Orthopaedic and Sports Physical Therapy*, **9**, 86-93.

Hanten, W.P., & Ramberg, C.L. (1988). Effect of stabilization on maximal isokinetic torque of the quadriceps femoris muscle during concentric and eccentric contractions. *Physical Therapy*, **68**, 219-222.

Harding, B., Black, T., Bruulsema, A., Maxwell, B., & Stratford, P. (1988). Reliability of a reciprocal test protocol performed on the kinetic communicator: An isokinetic test of knee extensor and flexor strength. *Journal of Orthopaedic and Sports Physical Therapy*, **10**, 218-223.

Harter, R.A., Osternig, L.R., Singer, K.M., James, S.L., Larson, R.L., & Jones, D.C. (1988). Long-term evaluation of knee stability and function following surgical reconstruction for anterior cruciate ligament insufficiency. *American Journal of Sports Medicine*, **16**, 434-443.

Harter, R.A., Osternig, L.R., & Standifer, L.W. (1990). Isokinetic evaluation of quadriceps and hamstrings symmetry following anterior cruciate ligament reconstruction. *Archives of Physical Medicine and Rehabilitation*, **71**, 465-468.

Hasue, M., Fujiwara, M., & Kikuchi, S. (1980). A new method of quantitative measurement of abdominal and back muscle strength. *Spine*, **5**, 143-148.

Haymes, E.M., & Dickinson, A.L. (1980). Characteristics of elite male and female ski racers. *Medicine and Science in Sports and Exercise*, **12**, 153-158.

Hellwig, E.V., & Perrin, D.H. (1991). A comparison of two positions for assessing shoulder rotator peak torque: The traditional frontal plane versus the plane of the scapula. *Isokinetics and Exercise Science*, **1**, 1-5.

Hester, J.R., & Falkel, F.E. (1984). Isokinetic evaluation of tibial rotation: Assessment of a stabilization technique. *Journal of Orthopaedic and Sports Physical Therapy*, **6**, 46-51.

Highgenboten, C.L., Jackson, A.W., & Meske, N.B. (1988). Concentric and eccentric torque comparisons for knee extension and flexion in young adult males and females using the kinetic communicator. *American Journal of Sports Medicine*, **16**, 234-237.

Hill, A.V. (1938). The heat of shortening and the dynamic constants of muscle. *Proceedings of the Royal Society of London (Biology)*, **126**, 136-195.

Hinson, M.N., Smith, W.C., & Funk, S. (1979). Isokinetics: A clarification. *Research Quarterly*, **50**, 30-35.

Hinton, R.Y. (1988). Isokinetic evaluation of shoulder rotational strength in high school baseball pitchers. *American Journal of Sports Medicine*, **16**, 274-279.

Hislop, H., & Perrine, J.J. (1967). The isokinetic concept of exercise. *Physical Therapy*, **47**, 114-117.

Holmes, J.R., & Alderink, G.J. (1984). Isokinetic strength characteristics of the quadriceps femoris and hamstring muscles in high school students. *Physical Therapy*, **64**, 914-918.

Hortobagyi, T., & Katch, F.I. (1990). Eccentric and concentric torque-velocity relationships during arm flexion and extension. *European Journal of Applied Physiology*, **60**, 395-401.

Housh, T.J., Thorland, W.G., Tharp, G.D., Johnson, G.O., & Cisar, C.J. (1984). Isokinetic leg flexion and extension strength of elite adolescent female track and field athletes. *Research Quarterly for Exercise and Sport*, **55**, 347-350.

Ivey, F.M., Calhoun, J.H., Rusche, K., & Bierschenk, J. (1985). Isokinetic testing of shoulder strength: Normal values. *Archives of Physical Medicine and Rehabilitation*, **66**, 384-386.

Jensen, R.C., Warren, B., Laursen, C., & Morrissey, M.C. (1991). Static pre-load effect on knee extensor isokinetic concentric and eccentric performance. *Medicine and Science in Sports and Exercise*, **23**, 10-14.

Jobe, F.W., Radovich Moynes, D., Tibone, J.E., & Perry, J. (1984). An EMG analysis of the shoulder in pitching—A second report. *American Journal of Sports Medicine*, **12**, 218-220.

Jobe, F.W., Tibone, J.E., Perry, J., & Moynes, D. (1983). An EMG analysis of the shoulder in throwing and pitching—A preliminary report. *American Journal of Sports Medicine*, **11**, 3-5.

Johnson, D. (1982). Controlling anterior shear during isokinetic knee extension exercise. *Journal of Orthopaedic and Sports Physical Therapy*, **4**, 23-31.

Johnson, J., & Siegel, D. (1978). Reliability of an isokinetic movement of the knee extensors. *Research Quarterly*, **49**, 88-90.

Johnston, T.B. (1937). The movements of the shoulder-joint—A plea for the use of the "plane of the scapula" as the plane of reference for movements occurring at the humero-scapular joint. *British Journal of Surgery*, **25**, 252-260.

Kannus, P. (1988a). Isokinetic peak torque and work relationship in the laterally unstable knee. *Canadian Journal of Sport Sciences*, **14**, 17-20.

Kannus, P. (1988b). Peak torque and total work relationship in the thigh muscles after anterior cruciate ligament injury. *Journal of Orthopaedic and Sports Physical Therapy*, **10**, 97-101.

Kannus, P. (1988c). Ratio of hamstring to quadriceps femoris muscles' strength in the anterior cruciate ligament insufficient knee. *Physical Therapy*, **68**, 961-965.

Kannus, P. (1988d). Relationship between peak torque and total work in an isokinetic contraction of the medial collateral ligament insufficient knee. *International Journal of Sports Medicine*, **9**, 294-296.

Kannus, P. (1991). Relationship between peak torque and angle-specific torques in an isokinetic contraction of normal and laterally unstable knee. *Journal of Orthopaedic and Sports Physical Therapy*, **13**, 89-94.

Kannus, P., Cook, L., & Alosa, D. (1992). Absolute and relative endurance parameters in isokinetic tests of muscular performance. *Journal of Sport Rehabilitation*, **1**, 2-12.

Kannus, P., & Jarvinen, M. (1989). Prediction of torque acceleration energy and power of thigh muscles from peak torque. *Medicine and Science in Sports and Exercise*, **21**, 304-307.

Kannus, P., & Kaplan, M. (1991). Angle-specific torques of thigh muscles: Variability analysis in 200 healthy adults. *Canadian Journal of Sport Sciences*, **16**, 264-270.

Kannus, P., & Yasuda, K. (1992). Value of isokinetic angle-specific torque measurements in normal and injured knees. *Medicine and Science in Sports and Exercise*, **24**, 292-297.

Karnofel, H., Wilkinson, K., & Lentell, G. (1989). Reliability of isokinetic muscle testing at the ankle. *Journal of Orthopaedic and Sports Physical Therapy*, **11**, 150-154.

Kaufman, K.R., An, K-N, Litchy, W.J., Morrey, B.F., & Chao, E.Y.S. (1991). Dynamic joint forces during knee isokinetic exercise. *American Journal of Sports Medicine*, **19**(3), 305-316.

Kendall, F.P., & McCreary, E.K. (1983). *Muscles: Testing and function.* Baltimore: Williams & Wilkins.

Klopfer, D.A., & Greij, S.D. (1988). Examining quadriceps/hamstrings performance at high velocity isokinetics in untrained subjects. *Journal of Orthopaedic and Sports Physical Therapy*, **10**, 18-22.

Knapik, J.J., Bauman, C.L., Jones, B.H., Harris, J.M., & Vaughan, L. (1991). Preseason strength and flexibility imbalances associated with athletic injuries in female collegiate athletes. *American Journal of Sports Medicine*, **19**, 76-81.

Knoeppel, D.E. (1985a). Alternative Cybex exercise positions. *Journal of Orthopaedic and Sports Physical Therapy*, **7**, 73-76.

Knoeppel, D.E. (1985b). Exercising isokinetically: Seated shoulder variations. *Journal of Orthopaedic and Sports Physical Therapy*, **7**, 124-126.

Kramer, J.F. (1990). Reliability of knee extensor and flexor torques during continuous concentric-eccentric cycles. *Archives of Physical Medicine and Rehabilitation*, **71**, 460-464.

Kramer, J.F., Vaz, M.D., & Hakansson, D. (1991). Effect of activation force on knee extensor torques. *Medicine and Science in Sports and Exercise*, **23**, 231-237.

Kues, J.M., Rothstein, J.M., & Lamb, R.L. (1992). Obtaining reliable measurements of knee extensor torque produced during maximal voluntary contractions: An experimental investigation. *Physical Therapy*, **72**, 492-501.

Langrana, N.A., & Lee, C.K. (1984). Isokinetic evaluation of trunk muscles. *Spine*, **9**, 171-175.

Langrana, N.A., Lee, C.K., Alexander, H., & Mayott, C.W. (1984). Quantitative assessment of back strength using isokinetic testing. *Spine*, **9**, 287-290.

Lavin, R.P., & Gross, M.T. (1990). Comparison of Johnson anti-shear accessory and standard dynamometer attachment for anterior and posterior tibial translation during isometric muscle contractions. *Journal of Orthopaedic and Sports Physical Therapy*, **11**, 547-553.

Lentell, G.L., Cashman, P.A., Shiomoto, K.J., & Spry, J.T. (1988). The effect of knee position on torque output during inversion and eversion movements at the ankle. *Journal of Orthopaedic and Sports Physical Therapy*, **10**, 177-183.

Lephart, S.M., Perrin, D.H., Fu, F.H., Gieck, J.C., McCue, F.C., & Irrgang, J.J. (1992). Relationship between selected physical characteristics and functional capacity in the anterior cruciate ligament–insufficient athlete. *Journal of Orthopaedic and Sports Physical Therapy*, **16**, 174-181.

Lephart, S.M., Perrin, D.H., Minger, K., & Fu, F.H. (1991). Sports specific functional tests for the anterior cruciate ligament insufficient athlete. *Athletic Training*, **26**, 44-50.

Leslie, M., Zachazewski, J., & Browne, P. (1990). Reliability of isokinetic torque values for ankle invertors and evertors. *Journal of Orthopaedic and Sports Physical Therapy*, **11**, 612-616.

Lesmes, G.R., Costill, D.L., Coyle, E.F., & Fink, W.J. (1978). Muscle strength and power changes during maximal isokinetic training. *Medicine and Science in Sports*, **10**, 266-269.

Levine, D., Klein, A., & Morrissey, M. (1991). Reliability of isokinetic concentric closed kinematic chain testing of the hip and knee extensors. *Isokinetics and Exercise Science*, **1**, 146-152.

Lucca, J.A., & Kline, K.K. (1989). Effects of upper and lower limb preference on torque production in the knee flexors and extensors. *Journal of Orthopaedic and Sports Physical Therapy*, **11**, 202-207.

Mayer, T.G., Smith, S.S., Kondraske, G., Gatchel, R.J., Carmichael, T.W., & Mooney, V. (1985). Quantification of lumbar function part 3: Preliminary data on isokinetic torso rotation testing with myoelectric spectral analysis in normal and low-back pain subjects. *Spine*, **10**, 912-920.

McGorry, R. (1989). Active dynamometry in quantitative evaluation and rehabilitation of musculoskeletal dysfunction. *Assistive Technology*, **1**, 91-99.

McMaster, W.C., Long, S.C., & Caiozzo, V.J. (1991). Isokinetic torque imbalances in the rotator cuff of the elite water polo player. *American Journal of Sports Medicine*, **19**, 72-75.

McMaster, W.C., Long, S.C., & Caiozzo, V.J. (1992). Shoulder torque changes in the swimming athlete. *American Journal of Sports Medicine*, **20**, 323-327.

Molczyk, L., Thigpen, L.K., Eickoff, J., Goldgar, D., & Gallagher, J.C. (1991). Reliability of testing the knee extensors and flexors in healthy adult women using a Cybex II isokinetic dynamometer. *Journal of Orthopaedic and Sports Physical Therapy*, **14**, 37-41.

Montgomery, L.C., Douglass, L.W., & Deuster, P.A. (1989). Reliability of an isokinetic test of muscle strength and endurance. *Journal of Orthopaedic and Sports Physical Therapy*, **10**, 315-322.

Morris, A., Lussier, L., Bell, G., & Dooley, J. (1983). Hamstring/quadriceps strength ratios in collegiate middle-distance and distance runners. *The Physician and Sportsmedicine*, **11**(10), 71-77.

Morrissey, M.C. (1987). The relationship between peak torque and work of the quadriceps and hamstrings after meniscectomy. *Journal of Orthopaedic and Sports Physical Therapy*, **8**, 405-408.

Negus, R.A., Rippe, J.M., Freedson, P., & Michaels, J. (1987). Heart rate, blood pressure, and oxygen consumption during orthopaedic rehabilitation exercise. *Journal of Orthopaedic and Sports Physical Therapy*, **8**, 346-350.

Nelson, S.G., & Duncan, P.W. (1983). Correction of isokinetic and isometric torque recordings for the effects of gravity. *Physical Therapy*, **63**, 674-676.

Nicholas, J.J., Robinson, L.R., Logan, A., & Robertson, R. (1989). Isokinetic testing in young nonathletic able-bodied subjects. *Archives of Physical Medicine and Rehabilitation*, **70**, 210-213.

Nisell, R., Ericson, M.O., Nemeth, G., & Ekholm, J. (1989). Tibiofemoral joint forces during isokinetic knee extension. *American Journal of Sports Medicine*, **17**, 49-54.

Oberg, B., Bergman, T., & Tropp, H. (1987). Testing of isokinetic muscle strength in the ankle. *Medicine and Science in Sports and Exercise*, **19**, 318-322.

Oberg, B., Moller, M., Gillquist, J., & Ekstrand, J. (1986). Isokinetic torque levels for knee extensors and knee flexors in soccer players. *International Journal of Sports Medicine*, **7**, 50-53.

Osternig, L.R., Bates, B.T., & James, S.L. (1980). Patterns of tibial rotary torque in knees of healthy subjects. *Medicine and Science in Sports and Exercise*, **12**, 195-199.

Osternig, L.R., Hamill, J., Lander, J.E., & Robertson, R. (1986). Co-activation of sprinter and distance runner muscles in isokinetic exercise. *Medicine and Science in Sports and Exercise*, **18**(4), 431-435.

Otis, J.C., Warren, R.F., Backus, S.I., Santner, T.J., & Mabrey, J.D. (1990). Torque production in the shoulder of the normal young adult male. *American Journal of Sports Medicine*, **18**, 119-123.

Pappas, A.M., Zawacki, R.M., & Sullivan, T.J. (1985). Biomechanics of baseball pitching: A preliminary report. *American Journal of Sports Medicine*, **13**, 216-222.

Patterson, L.A., & Spivey, W.E. (1992). Validity and reliability of the LIDO active isokinetic system. *Journal of Orthopaedic and Sports Physical Therapy*, **15**, 32-36.

Pawlowski, D., & Perrin, D.H. (1989). Relationship between shoulder and elbow isokinetic peak torque, torque acceleration energy, average power, and total work and throwing velocity in intercollegiate pitchers. *Athletic Training*, **24**, 129-132.

Peel, C., & Alland, M.J. (1990). Cardiovascular responses to isokinetic trunk exercise. *Physical Therapy*, **70**, 503-510.

Perrin, D.H. (1986). Reliability of isokinetic measures. *Athletic Training*, **10**, 319-321.

Perrin, D.H., Haskvitz, E.M., & Weltman, A. (1991). Effect of gravity correction on isokinetic average force of the quadriceps and hamstring muscle groups in women runners. *Isokinetics and Exercise Science*, **1**, 99-102.

Perrin, D.H., Hellwig, E.V., Tis, L.L., & Shenk, B.S. (1992). Effect of gravity correction on shoulder rotation isokinetic average force and reciprocal muscle group ratios. *Isokinetics and Exercise Science*, **2**, 30-33.

Perrin, D.H., Lephart, S.M., & Weltman, A. (1989). Specificity of training on computer obtained isokinetic measures. *Journal of Orthopaedic and Sports Physical Therapy*, **10**, 495-498.

Perrin, D.H., Robertson, R.J., & Ray, R.L. (1987). Bilateral isokinetic peak torque, torque acceleration energy, power, and work relationships in athletes and nonathletes. *Journal of Orthopaedic and Sports Physical Therapy*, **9**, 184-189.

Perrin, D.H., Tis, L.L., Hellwig, E.V., & Shenk, B.S. (in press). Relationship between isokinetic average force, peak force, average torque, and peak torque of the shoulder internal and external rotator muscle groups. *Isokinetics and Exercise Science*.

Peter, J.B., Barnard, R.J., Edgerton, V.R., Gillespie, C.A., & Stempel, K.E. (1972). Metabolic profiles of three fiber types of skeletal muscle in guinea pigs and rabbits. *Biochemistry*, **11**, 2627-2633.

Petersen, S., Wessel, J., Bagnall, K., Wilkins, H., Quinney, A., & Wenger, H. (1990). Influence of concentric resistance training on concentric and eccentric strength. *Archives of Physical Medicine and Rehabilitation*, **71**, 101-105.

Poulmedis, P. (1985). Isokinetic maximal torque power of Greek elite soccer players. *Journal of Orthopaedic and Sports Physical Therapy*, **6**, 293-295.

Rasch, P.J. (1989). *Kinesiology and applied anatomy*. Philadelphia: Lea & Febiger.

Rasch, P.J., & Burke, R.K. (1978). *Kinesiology and applied anatomy*. Philadelphia: Lea & Febiger.

Richter, K.J. (1992). Subcutaneous hemorrhage in a patient on coumadin: An isokinetic exercise complication. *Journal of Sport Rehabilitation*, **1**, 264-266.

Rothstein, J.M., Delitto, A., Sinacore, D.R., & Rose, S.J. (1983). Electromyographic, peak torque, and power relationships during isokinetic movement. *Physical Therapy*, **63**, 926-933.

Rothstein, J.M., Lamb, R.L., & Mayhew, T.P. (1987). Clinical uses of isokinetic measurements. *Physical Therapy*, **67**, 1840-1844.

Ryan, L.M., Magidow, P.S., & Duncan, P.W. (1991). Velocity-specific and mode-specific effects of eccentric isokinetic training of the hamstrings. *Journal of Orthopaedic and Sports Physical Therapy*, **13**, 33-39.

Safrit, M.J., & Wood, T.M. (Eds.) (1989). *Measurement concepts in physical education and exercise science*. Champaign, IL: Human Kinetics.

Sapega, A.A., Nicholas, J.A., Sokolow, D., & Saraniti, A. (1982). The nature of torque "overshoot" in Cybex isokinetic dynamometry. *Medicine and Science in Sports and Exercise*, **14**(5), 368-375.

Schlinkman, B. (1984). Norms for high school football players derived from Cybex data reduction computer. *Journal of Orthopaedic and Sports Physical Therapy*, **5**, 243-245.

Seger, J.Y., Westing, S.H., Hanson, M., Karlson, E., Ekblom, B. (1988). A new dynamometer measuring concentric and eccentric muscle strength in accelerated, decelerated, or isokinetic movements. *European Journal of Applied Physiology*, **57**, 526-530.

Seto, J.L., Orofino, A.S., Morrissey, M.C., Medeiros, J.M., & Mason, W.J. (1988). Assessment of quadriceps/hamstring strength, knee ligament stability, functional and sports activity levels five years after anterior cruciate ligament reconstruction. *American Journal of Sports Medicine*, **16**, 170-180.

Seymour, R.J., & Bacharach, D.W. (1990). The effect of position and speed on ankle plantar flexion in females. *Journal of Orthopaedic and Sports Physical Therapy*, **12**, 153-156.

Sherman, W.M., Pearson, D.R., Plyley, M.J., Costill, D.L., Habansky, A.J., & Vogelgesang, D.A. (1982). Isokinetic rehabilitation after surgery. *American Journal of Sports Medicine*, **10**, 155-161.

Sinacore, D.R., Rothstein, J.M., Delitto, A., & Rose, S.J. (1983). Effect of damp on isokinetic measurements. *Physical Therapy*, **63**, 1248-1250.

Smidt, G., Herring, T., Amundsen, L., Rogers, M., Russell, A., & Lehmann, T. (1983). Assessment of abdominal and back extensor function: A quantitative approach and results for chronic low-back patients. *Spine*, **8**, 211-219.

Smith, D.J., Quinney, H.A., & Steadward, R.D. (1982). Physiological profiles of the Canadian Olympic hockey team (1980). *Canadian Journal of Applied Sport Sciences*, **7**, 142-146.

Smith, D.J., Quinney, H.A., Wenger, H.A., Steadward, R.D., & Sexsmith, J.R. (1981). Isokinetic torque outputs of professional and elite amateur ice hockey players. *Journal of Orthopaedic and Sports Physical Therapy*, **3**, 42-47.

Smith, S.S., Mayer, T.G., Gatchel, R.J., & Becker, T.J. (1985). Quantification of lumbar function. *Spine*, **10**, 757-764.

Soderberg, G.J., & Blaschak, M.J. (1987). Shoulder internal and external rotation peak torque production through a velocity spectrum in differing positions. *Journal of Orthopaedic and Sports Physical Therapy*, **8**, 518-524.

Stafford, M.G., & Grana, W.A. (1984). Hamstring/quadriceps ratios in college football players: A high velocity evaluation. *American Journal of Sports Medicine*, **12**, 209-211.

Stauber, W.T. (1989a). Eccentric action of muscles: Physiology, injury, and adaptations. In K.B. Pandolph (Ed.), *Exercise and sports sciences review* (pp. 157-185). Baltimore: Williams & Wilkins.

Stauber, W.T. (1989b). Measurement of muscle function in man. In V. Grisogono (Ed.), *Sports injuries* (pp. 187-212). New York: Churchill Livingstone.

Stratford, P.W., Bruulsema, A., Maxwell, B., Black, T., & Harding, B. (1990). The effect of inter-trial rest interval on the assessment of isokinetic thigh muscle torque. *Journal of Orthopaedic and Sports Physical Therapy*, **11**, 362-366.

Tabin, G.C., Gregg, J.R., & Bonci, T. (1985). Predictive leg strength values in immediately prepubescent and postpubescent athletes. *American Journal of Sports Medicine*, **13**, 387-389.

Taylor, N.A.S., Sanders, R.H., Howick, E.I., & Stanley, S.N. (1991). Static and dynamic assessment of the Biodex dynamometer. *European Journal of Applied Physiology*, **62**, 180-188.

Tesch, P.A. (1983). Physiological characteristics of elite kayak paddlers. *Canadian Journal of Applied Sport Sciences*, **8**, 87-91.

Thigpen, L.K., Blanke, D., & Lang, P. (1990). The reliability of two different Cybex isokinetic systems. *Journal of Orthopaedic and Sports Physical Therapy*, **12**, 157-162.

Thistle, H.G., Hislop, H.J., Moffroid, M., & Lohman, E.W. (1967). Isokinetic contraction: A new concept of resistive exercise. *Archives of Physical Medicine and Rehabilitation*, **48**, 279-282.

Thomas, L.E. (1984). Isokinetic torque levels for adult females: Effects of age and body size. *Journal of Orthopaedic and Sports Physical Therapy*, **6**, 21-24.

Thompson, N.N., Gould, J.A., Davies, G.J., Ross, D.E., & Price, S. (1985). Descriptive measures of isokinetic trunk testing. *Journal of Orthopaedic and Sports Physical Therapy*, **7**, 43-49.

Thorstensson, A., & Arvidson, A. (1982). Trunk muscle strength and low back pain. *Scandinavian Journal of Rehabilitation Medicine*, **14**, 69-75.

Thorstensson, A., & Karlsson, J. (1976). Fatiguability and fibre composition of human skeletal muscle. *Acta Physiologica Scandinavica*, **98**, 318-322.

Thorstensson, A., & Nilsson, J. (1982). Trunk muscle strength during constant velocity movements. *Scandinavian Journal of Rehabilitation Medicine*, **14**, 61-68.

Timm, K.E. (1986). Validation of the Johnson anti-shear accessory as an accurate and effective clinical isokinetic instrument. *Journal of Orthopaedic and Sports Physical Therapy*, **7**, 298-303.

Tippett, S.R. (1986). Lower extremity strength and active range of motion in college baseball pitchers: A comparison between stance leg and kick leg. *Journal of Orthopaedic and Sports Physical Therapy*, **8**, 10-14.

Tis, L.L., Perrin, D.H., Snead, D.B., & Weltman, A. (1991). Isokinetic strength of the trunk and hip in female runners. *Isokinetics and Exercise Science*, **1**, 22-25.

Tis, L.L., Perrin, D.H., Weltman, A., Ball, D., & Gieck, J.H. (1992). *The effect of preload and range of motion on average and peak torque of the knee extensor and flexor musculature.* Manuscript submitted for publication.

Tomberlin, J.P., Basford, J.R., Schwen, E.E., Orte, P.A., Scott, S.G., Laughman, R.K., & Ilstrup, D.M. (1991). Comparative study of isokinetic eccentric and concentric quadriceps training. *Journal of Orthopaedic and Sports Physical Therapy*, **14**, 31-36.

Tredinnick, T.J., & Duncan, P.W. (1988). Reliability of measurements of concentric and eccentric isokinetic loading. *Physical Therapy*, **68**, 656-659.

VanSwearingen, J.M. (1983). Measuring wrist muscle strength. *Journal of Orthopaedic and Sports Physical Therapy*, **4**, 217-228.

Walmsley, R.P., & Szybbo, C. (1987). A comparative study of the torque generated by the shoulder internal and external rotator muscles in different positions and at varying speeds. *Journal of Orthopaedic and Sports Physical Therapy*, **9**, 217-222.

Watkins, M.P., Harris, B.A., Wender, S., Zarins, B., & Rowe, C.R. (1983). Effect of patellectomy on the function of the quadriceps and hamstrings. *Journal of Bone and Joint Surgery*, **65-A**, 390-395.

Weir, J.P., Wagner, L.L., Housh, T.J., & Johnson, G.O. (1992). Horizontal abduction and adduction strength at the shoulder of high school wrestlers across age. *Journal of Orthopaedic and Sports Physical Therapy*, **15**, 183-186.

Weltman, A., Tippett, S., Janney, C., Strand, K., Rians, C., Cahill, B.R., & Katch, F.I. (1988). Measurement of isokinetic strength in prepubertal males. *Journal of Orthopaedic and Sports Physical Therapy*, **9**, 345-351.

Wennerberg, D. (1991). Reliability of an isokinetic dorsiflexion and plantar flexion apparatus. *American Journal of Sports Medicine*, **19**, 519-522.

Westing, S.H., Cresswell, A.G., & Thorstensson, A. (1991). Muscle activation during maximal voluntary eccentric and concentric knee extension. *European Journal of Applied Physiology*, **62**, 104-108.

Westing, S.H., & Seger, J.Y. (1989). Eccentric and concentric torque-velocity characteristics, torque output comparisons, and gravity effect torque corrections for the quadriceps and hamstring muscles in females. *International Journal of Sports Medicine*, **10**, 175-180.

Westing, S.H., Seger, J.Y., Karlson, E., & Ekblom, B. (1988). Eccentric and concentric torque-velocity characteristics of the quadriceps femoris in man. *European Journal of Applied Physiology*, **58**, 100-104.

Westing, S.H., Seger, J.Y., & Thorstensson, A. (1990). Effects of electrical stimulation on eccentric and concentric torque-velocity relationships during knee extension in man. *Acta Physiologica Scandinavica*, **140**, 17-22.

Westing, S.H., Seger, J.Y., & Thorstensson, A. (1991). Isoacceleration: A new concept of resistive exercise. *Medicine and Science in Sports and Exercise*, **23**, 631-635.

Wilhite, M.R., Cohen, E.R., & Wilhite, S.C. (1992). Reliability of concentric and eccentric measurements of quadriceps performance using the Kin-Com dynamometer: The effect of testing order for three different speeds. *Journal of Orthopaedic and Sports Physical Therapy*, **15**, 175-182.

Winter, D.A., Wells, R.P., & Orr, G.W. (1981). Errors in the use of isokinetic dynamometers. *European Journal of Applied Physiology*, **46**, 397-408.

Wong, D.L.K., Glasheen-Wray, M., & Andrews, L.F. (1984). Isokinetic evaluation of the ankle invertors and evertors. *Journal of Orthopaedic and Sports Physical Therapy*, **5**, 246-252.

Woodhouse, M.L., Heinen, J.R.K., Shall, L., & Bragg, K. (1990). Isokinetic trunk rotation parameters of athletes utilizing lumber/sacral supports. *Athletic Training*, **25**, 240-243.

Worrell, T.W., Denegar, C.R., Armstrong, S.L., & Perrin, D.H. (1990). Effect of body position on hamstring muscle group average torque. *Journal of Orthopaedic and Sports Physical Therapy*, **11**, 449-451.

Worrell, T.W., Perrin, D.H., & Denegar, C.R. (1989). The influence of hip position on quadriceps and hamstring peak torque and reciprocal muscle group ratio values. *Journal of Orthopaedic and Sports Physical Therapy*, **11**, 104-107.

Worrell, T.W., Perrin, D.H., Gansneder, B.M., & Gieck, J.H. (1991). Comparison of isokinetic strength and flexibility measures between hamstring injured and non-injured athletes. *Journal of Orthopaedic and Sports Physical Therapy*, **13**, 118-125.

Wyatt, M.P., & Edwards, A.M. (1981). Comparison of quadriceps and hamstring torque values during isokinetic exercise. *Journal of Orthopaedic and Sports Physical Therapy*, **3**, 48-56.

Index